Respiratory
Home Exercise Guide & Workbook

Plus
Exercise Benefits & Precautions

Lost Temple Fitness & Rehab

Karen Cutler: LPTA, ACE Certified Personal Trainer,
Medical, Cancer, Arthritis & Therapeutic Exercise Specialist

It is advised that you always check with your medical doctor or physical therapist before starting an exercise program or change in diet.

Websites

LostTempleFitness.com
LostTempleCancer.com
LostTempleNutrition.com
LostTemplePets.com
LostTempleArt.com

Introduction

It has been proven that exercise and nutrition are two of the main factors that you can control for a healthy lifestyle. Many people do not know how to start or progress an exercise program. There are hundreds of pictures for beginner, intermediate and advanced exercise programs, as well as a list of equipment that you can use in the home. This also includes worksheets to help you track your exercises and progress.

The respiratory section includes information on each disease, exercises that should be done for each health condition, as well as precautions and contraindications. Some of these diseases include, but not limited to COPD, Asthma, Bronchitis, Cystic Fibrosis, Idiopathic Pulmonary Fibrosis, as well as Oxygen Therapy.

This book is for:

- Those with a history of respiratory disease to be used in conjunction with a physician or other health care provider and/or physical therapist recommendations.
- The beginner who has never exercised before.
- The individual that has mastered the basics but wants to know how to advance to the next level.
- Pre/post rehab individuals who would like to advance or want a list of exercise programs to follow.
- The personal trainer, physical therapist, or other coaches who would like their client to have a list of exercises that can be progressed or know more about precautions with clients or patients with pulmonary disease.

This book is NOT for or may need modification:

- Chronic or acute disorders/injury's that is not being followed by a health care professional. This book can be used in conjunction with a rehab program.
- If you are over 40 and have never exercised before, it is advised that a physician clears you first.
- Undiagnosed pain.
- The person that does not feel they can safely modify their individual program, although can be used in conjunction with rehab or coaches/personal trainers.
- People with the following issues that have not been cleared by an MD for an exercise program or in conjunctionwith rehab. These issues may be addressed in future volumes: Arthritis, Cardiac disease, Cancer or Diabetes.

What is covered in this book?

Respiratory Disease, including:
- o Description
- o Signs/Symptoms
- o Treatment
- o Exercise
- COPD
- Asthma
- Bronchitis
- Cystic Fibrosis
- Idiopathic Pulmonary Fibrosis
- Oxygen Therapy

- Home Exercise Programs – pictures with explanations and worksheets
    - o Myofascial release
    - o Flexibility – Stretching
    - o Core Stability
    - o Balance with progression to Standing Strengthening exercises
    - o Strengthening
        - Lower extremity - Lying and Seated
        - Upper extremity
- Benefits and Factors to consider before starting an exercise program
- Vital signs and how to monitor exercise intensity
- Temperature – Heat and Cold
- Dehydration
- Equipment needed for home exercise
- Warm up/cool down
- Duration, Frequency, Intensity and Primary Movement Patterns
- Anatomy
- Self-Tests

It is advised that you always check with your medical doctor or physical therapist before starting an exercise program or change in diet.

LOST TEMPLE FITNESS & REHAB

INTRODUCTION

Respiratory
See Section for Specific TOC

REFERENCES

HOME EXERCISE PROGRAM
See Section for Specific TOC

REFERENCES

Respiratory Disease and Exercise

It is beneficial for people who have a history or are currently undergoing treatment for respiratory disease to engage inan exercise program. This book is for educational purposes and should not be substituted for the direction of a physician or other healthcare provider (*see Disclaimer above*). Before starting an exercise program, especially if you have a history of respiratory disease, you should consult with a physician and/or physical therapist.

Please read the 2nd section of this book to learn about precautions, even if you are a healthy individual and are reading this version to learn about preventing pulmonary disease. This includes education on how exercise can help with endurance, balance, muscle strengthening and flexibility.

Most of the respiratory research is from the:
CDC – Center for Disease Control and Prevention
NIH – National Heart, Blood and Lung Institute (unless otherwise specified)

Please see *Respiratory References* for links.

This book is not meant to substitute an exercise program prescribed by a health care professional but designed to accompany their recommendations. Please consult with your physician before starting any exercise program.

Who is this section recommended for?

- Those with a history of pulmonary disease to be used in conjunction with the physician, respiratory therapist orother health care provider and/or physical therapist recommendations.
- The average adult looking to reduce their risks of pulmonary disease.
- Patients currently undergoing Pulmonary Rehab to be used in conjunction with a respiratory therapist, healthcare provider and/or physical therapist recommendations.
- Physical therapists and other health care providers to be used to prescribe a home exercise program.

Who is this section not for?
- Those who are not able to follow or modify a program without supervision.
- Those who have other medical issues, such as cancer, fracture risks or other acute/chronic issues that have not been cleared by an MD.

What is covered in this section?
Respiratory Disease, including:
- Description
- Signs/Symptoms
- Treatment
- Exercise
    - COPD
    - Asthma
    - Bronchitis
    - Cystic Fibrosis
    - Idiopathic Pulmonary Fibrosis
    - Oxygen Therapy

Quick Summary this Section

Chronic Obstructive Pulmonary Disease (COPD)
- COPD, or chronic obstructive pulmonary disease, is a progressive disease that makes it hard to breathe.
- COPD includes chronic bronchitis and emphysema
- Signs, symptoms and complications
- Treatments
- Medications
- Managing COPD
- Exercise
- Exercise Precautions

Asthma
- A chronic lung disease that inflames and narrows the airways.
- Common Signs and Symptoms
- Control and Treatment
- Diet
- Medications
- Exercise

Bronchitis
- Acute vs Chronic
- Signs, Symptoms, and Complications
- Treatment
- Exercise

Cystic Fibrosis
- Cystic fibrosis, or CF, is an inherited disease of the secretory glands. Secretory glands include glands that make mucus and sweat.
- Signs, Symptoms, and Complications
- Treatment
- Exercise

Idiopathic Pulmonary Fibrosis
- Pulmonary fibrosis is a disease in which tissue deep in your lungs becomes thick and stiff, or scarred, over time. The formation of scar tissue is called fibrosis.
- Signs, Symptoms, and Complications
- Treatment
- Life Changes
- Exercise & Breathing Exercises

Oxygen Therapy
- Oxygen therapy is a treatment that provides you with extra oxygen.
- Oxygen is a gas that your body needs to function. Normally, your lungs absorb oxygen from the air you breathe, but some conditions can prevent you from getting enough oxygen.

COPD - Chronic Obstructive Pulmonary Disease

COPD, or chronic obstructive pulmonary disease, is a progressive disease that makes it hard to breathe. Progressive means the disease gets worse over time.

- COPD can cause coughing that produces large amounts of a slimy substance called mucus, wheezing, shortness of breath, chest tightness, and other symptoms.
- Cigarette smoking is the leading cause of COPD. Most people who have COPD smoke or used to smoke, however, up to 25 percent of people with COPD never smoked.
- Long-term exposure to other lung irritants—such as air pollution, chemical fumes, or dusts—also may contribute to COPD.
- A rare genetic condition calledalpha-1 antitrypsin (AAT) deficiency can also cause the disease.

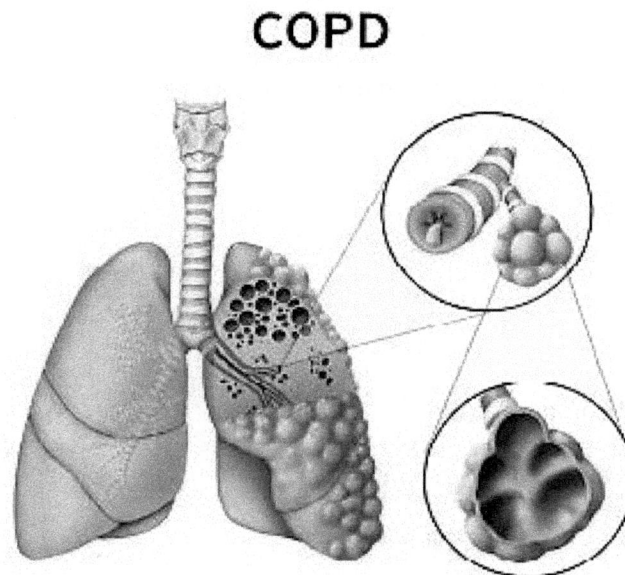

Overview

To understand COPD, it helps to understand how the lungs work. The air that you breathe goes down your windpipe into tubes in your lungs called bronchial tubes or airways.

- Within the lungs, your bronchial tubes branch many times into thousands of smaller, thinner tubes called bronchioles. These tubes end in bunches of tiny round air sacs called alveoli.
- Small blood vessels called capillaries run along the walls of the air sacs. When air reaches the air sacs, oxygen passes through the air sac walls into the blood in the capillaries.
- At the same time, a waste product, called carbon dioxide (CO_2) gas, moves from the capillaries into the air sacs. This process, called gas exchange, brings in oxygen for the body to use for vital functions and removes the CO_2.
- The airways and air sacs are elastic or stretchy. When you breathe in, each air sac fills up with air, like a small balloon. When you breathe out, the air sacs deflate, and the air goes out.

In COPD, less air flows in and out of the airways because of one or more of the following:

- The airways and air sacs lose their elastic quality.
- The walls between many of the air sacs are destroyed.
- The walls of the airways become thick and inflamed.
- The airways make more mucus than usual and can become clogged.

Emphysema and Chronic Bronchitis	In the United States, the term COPD includes two main conditions—**emphysema** and **chronic bronchitis.**
	
	• In **emphysema,** the walls between many of the air sacs are damaged. As a result, the air sacs lose their shapeand become floppy.
	    o This damage also can destroy the walls of the air sacs, leading to fewer and larger air sacs instead of many tiny ones.
	    o If this happens, the amount of gas exchange in the lungs is reduced.
	• In **chronic bronchitis**, the lining of the airways stays constantly irritated and inflamed, and this causes the lining to swell.
	    o Lots of thick mucus forms in the airways, making it hard to breathe.
	
	## Chronic Obstructive Pulmonary Disease
	Lorem ipsum dolor sit amet consectetur adipsicing elit
	
	Normal alveoli Emphysema
	
	Normal bronchus Bronchitis
	
	Most people who have COPD have both emphysema and chronic bronchitis, but the severity of each condition varies from person to person. Thus, the general term COPD is more accurate.

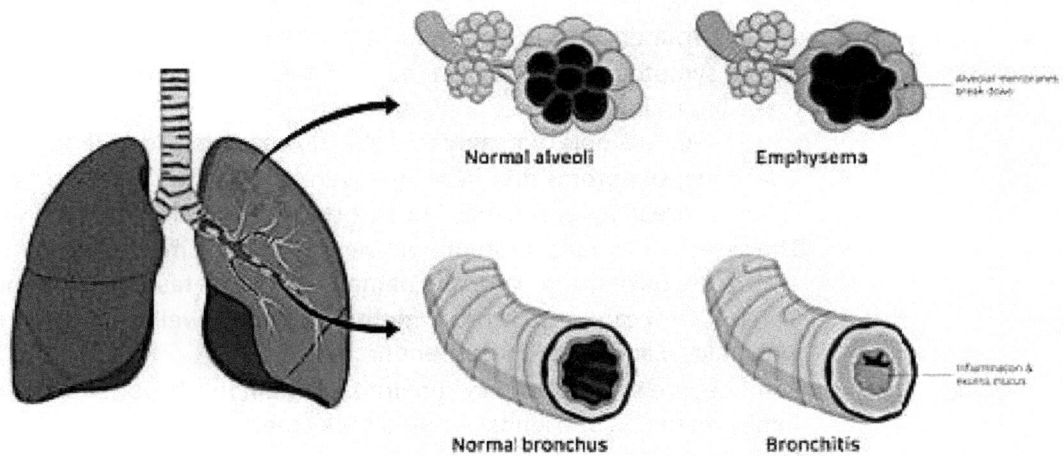

Signs, Symptoms, and Complications	At first, COPD may cause no symptoms or only mild symptoms. As the disease gets worse, symptoms usually become more severe.
	
	Common signs and symptoms of COPD include:
	• An ongoing cough or a cough that produces a lot of mucus; this is often called smoker's cough.
	• Shortness of breath, especially with physical activity
	• Wheezing or a whistling or squeaky sound when you breathe
	• Chest tightness
	
	If you have COPD, you also may often have colds or other respiratory infections such as the flu, or influenza.
	
	• Not everyone who has the symptoms described above has COPD. Likewise, not everyone who has COPD has these symptoms.
	   o Some of the symptoms of COPD are similar to the symptoms of other diseases and conditions.
	   o Your doctor can determine if you have COPD.
	• If your symptoms are mild, you may not notice them, or you may adjust your lifestyle to make breathing easier.
	   o For example, you may take the elevator instead of the stairs.
	• Over time, symptoms may become severe enough to cause you to see a doctor.
	   o Forexample, you may become short of breath during physical exertion.
	• The severity of your symptoms will depend on how much lung damage you have.
	   o If youkeep smoking, the damage will occur faster than if you stop smoking.
	• Severe COPD can cause other symptoms, such as swelling in your ankles, feet, or legs; weight loss; and lower muscle endurance.
	• Some severe symptoms may require treatment in a hospital. You—or, if you are unable, family members or friends—should seek emergency care if you are experiencing the following:
	   o You are having a hard time catching your breath or talking.
	   o Your lips or fingernails turn blue or gray, a sign of a low oxygen level in your blood.
	   o People around you notice that you are not mentally alert.
	   o Your heartbeat is very fast.
	   o The recommended treatment for symptoms that are getting worse is not working.

Treatments	**Lifestyle Changes**
	• Quitting smoking is the most important step you can take to treat COPD. Talk with your doctor about programs and products that can help you quit.
	• Try to avoid secondhand smoke and places with dusts, fumes, or other toxic substances that you may inhale.
	• If you have COPD, especially more severe forms, you may have trouble eating enough because of symptoms such as shortness of breath and fatigue. As a result, you may not get all the calories and nutrients you need, which can worsen your symptoms and raise your risk for infections.
	• Talk with your doctor about following an eating plan that will meet your nutritional needs. Your doctor may suggest eating smaller, more frequent meals; resting before eating; and taking vitamins or nutritional supplements.
	• Talk with your doctor about what types of activity are safe for you. You may find it hard to remain active with your symptoms. However, physical activity can strengthen the muscles that help you breathe and improve your overall wellness.
	
	Pulmonary Rehabilitation
	• Pulmonary rehabilitation or rehab is a broad program that helps improve the well-being of people who have chronic breathing problems.
	• Rehab may include an exercise program, disease management training, and nutritional and psychological counseling. The program's goal is to help you stay active and carry out your daily activities.
	• Your rehab team may include doctors, nurses, physical therapists, respiratory therapists, exercise specialists, and dietitians. These health professionals will create a program that meets your needs.
	
	Oxygen Therapy (also see *Oxygen Therapy* for more information)
	• If you have severe COPD and low levels of oxygen in your blood, oxygen therapy can help you breathe better. For this treatment, oxygen is delivered through nasal prongs or a mask.
	• You may need extra oxygen all the time or only at certain times. For some people who have severe COPD, using extra oxygen for most of the day can help them:
	   ○ Do tasks or activities while experiencing fewer symptoms
	   ○ Protect their hearts and other organs from damage
	   ○ Sleep more during the night and improve alertness during the day
	   ○ Live longer
	
	Surgery
	Surgery may benefit some people who have COPD. Surgery usually is a last resort for people who have severe symptoms that have not improved from taking medicines. Surgeries for people who have COPD that is mainly related to emphysema include bullectomy and lung volume reduction surgery (LVRS). A lung transplant might be an option for people who have very severe COPD.
	• BULLECTOMY - When the walls of the air sacs are destroyed, larger air spaces called bullae form. These air spaces can become so large that they interfere with breathing. In a bullectomy, doctors remove one or more very large bullae from the lungs.
	• LUNG VOLUME REDUCTION SURGERY - In LVRS, surgeons remove damaged tissue from the lungs. This helps the lungs work better. In carefully selected patients, LVRS can improve breathing and quality of life.
	• LUNG TRANSPLANT - During a lung transplant, doctors remove your damaged lung and replace it with a healthy lung from a donor. A lung transplant can improve your lung function and quality of life. However, lung transplants have many risks, such as infections and rejection of the transplanted lung.

Medicines	**BRONCHODILATORS**
	• Bronchodilators relax the muscles around your airways. This helps open your airways and makes breathing easier.
	• Depending on the severity of your COPD, your doctor may prescribe short-acting or long-acting bronchodilators.
	    o *Short-acting bronchodilators* last about 4–6 hours and should be used as needed.
	    o *Long-acting bronchodilators* last about 12 hours or more and are used every day.
	• Most bronchodilators are taken using a device called an inhaler. This device allows the medicine to go straight to your lungs. Not all inhalers are used the same way. Ask your health care providers to show you the correct way to use your inhaler.
	• If your COPD is mild, your doctor may only prescribe a short-acting inhaled bronchodilator. In this case, you may use the medicine only when symptoms occur.
	• If your COPD is moderate or severe, your doctor may prescribe regular treatment with short- and long-acting bronchodilators.

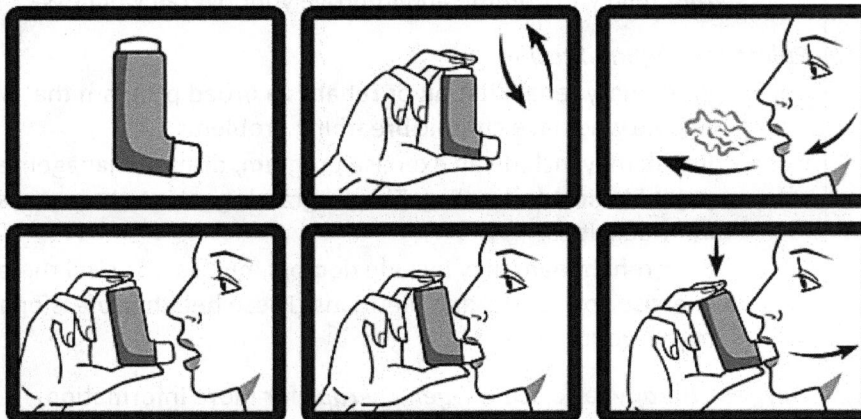

Combination Bronchodilators PLUS Inhaled Glucocorticosteroids (Steroids)
- In general, using inhaled steroids alone is not a preferred treatment.
  - If your COPD is moresevere, or if your symptoms flare up often, your doctor may prescribe a combination of medicines that includes a bronchodilator and an inhaled steroid.
  - Steroids help reduce airway inflammation.
- Your doctor may ask you to try inhaled steroids with the bronchodilator for a trial period of 6 weeks to 3 months to see whether the addition of the steroid helps relieve your breathing problems.

Managing COPD	**You can do things to help manage COPD and its symptoms.** For example: • Do activities slowly. • Put items you use often in one easy-to-reach place. • Find simple ways to cook, clean, and do other chores. For example, you might want to use a small table or cart with wheels tomove things around and a pole or tongs with long handles to reach things. • Ask for help in making things more accessible in your house so that you will not need to climb stairs as often. • Keep your clothes loose, and wear clothes and shoes that are easy to put on and take off.

Exercise
 	
(HealthLine and COPD Store)
	Different types of exercise can help COPD patients in different ways.
	For example:
	• **Cardiovascular exercise** involves steady aerobic activity that uses large muscle groups and strengthens your heart and lungs. This type of exercise improves your body's ability to use oxygen. Over time, you'll experience decreased heart rate and blood pressure and your heart won't need to work as hard during physical activities, which will improve your breathing.
	• **Strengthening or resistance exercises** use repeated muscle contractions to break down and then rebuild muscle. Resistance exercises for the upper body can help build strength in your respiratory muscles.
	• **Stretching and flexibility exercises** like yoga and Pilates can enhance coordination and breathing.
	
	What Type of Exercise You Should Do and Which Activities to Avoid
	
	Frequency
	• When exercising with COPD, it's important not to overdo it. Increase the amount of time you exercise very gradually. As a precursor to an exercise program, practice coordinating your breathing with daily activities. This can help strengthen postural muscles used for standing, sitting, and walking. From this base, you can begin to incorporate cardiovascular exercise into your routine.
	• Start out with modest exercise goals and build up slowly to a 20 to 30-minute session, three to four times each week. To do this, you can begin with a short walk and see how far you can go before you become breathless.
	• Whenever you start to feel short of breath, stop and rest.
	• Over time, you can set specific goals to increase your walking distance. Try an increase of 10 feet per day as your first goal.
	
	Exertion
	• Use a Rated Perceived Exertion (RPE) scale to measure the intensity of your exercise. This scale allows you to use numbers from 0 to 10 to rate the level of difficulty of a physical activity.
	   ○ For example, sitting in a chair would rate as level 0, or inactive.
	   ○ Taking an exercise stress test or performing a very difficult physical challenge would rate as level 10.
	   ○ On the RPE scale, level 3 is considered "moderate" and level 4 is described as "somewhat heavy."
	• People with COPD should exercise between levels 3 and 4 most of the time. Be aware that when you're using this scale, you should consider your level of fatigue and individual factors such as shortness of breath to prevent over-exertion.
	
	Breathing
	• Shortness of breath while working out means that your body needs more oxygen. You can restore oxygen to your system by slowing down your breathing.
	   ○ To breathe more slowly, focus on inhaling through your nose with your mouth closed, then exhaling through pursed lips.
	• This will warm, moisturize, and filter the air you breathe and allow for more complete lung action. To help decrease the rate of your breathing while you exercise, try making your exhalations twice as long as your inhalations.
	   ○ For example, if you inhale for two seconds, then exhale for four seconds.

Exercise Precautions *HealthLine* *and* *COPD Store*	Physical activity is an important part of managing your COPD, but you should take the following precautions to ensure safe exercise: • Do not work out in extreme temperatures. ○ Hot, cold, or humid conditions can affect your circulation, making breathing more difficult, and possibly causing chest pain. • Avoid hilly courses, as exercising on hills may lead to over-exertion. ○ If you must traverse ahilly area, slow your pace and monitor your heart rate closely, walking or stopping if needed. • Be sure to exhale when lifting any moderately heavy object. ○ In general, try to avoid liftingor pushing heavy objects. • If you become short of breath, dizzy, or weak during any activity, stop exercising and rest. ○ If symptoms continue, call your doctor. They might recommend changes to your medications, diet, or fluid intake before you continue your program. • Ask your doctor for guidance regarding your exercise program after you start new medications, as medicine can affect your response to activity. • Regular exercise has special challenges for those living with COPD, but the benefits can outweigh the difficulties. ○ By learning proper techniques and using precaution, physicalactivity can become one of the most important tools in your arsenal to manage your condition. *(HealthLine)* ***Signs You Should Stop Exercising*** *(COPD Store)* • It is important to listen to what your body is telling you, especially when exercising with COPD. • If you experience any of the following symptoms, you should immediately stop exercising and sit down with your feet elevated. • If you are still unable to regain control of them, call 9-1-1. • However, even if you do feel better, you should still report these symptoms to your doctor. ○ Experiencing Troubles Walking, Talking, or Thinking ○ Nausea ○ Dizziness ○ Lightheadedness ○ Irregular or Rapid Heart Rate ○ Overall Weakness ○ Extreme Shortness of Breath, Even After Taking Medications ○ Severe Pressure or Pain in Your Arms, Chest, Neck, Jaw, or Shoulder

Asthma

A chronic lung disease that inflames and narrows the airways.
- o Asthma causes recurring periods of wheezing (a whistling sound when you breathe), chest tightness, shortness of breath, and coughing.
- o The coughing often occurs at night or early in the morning.

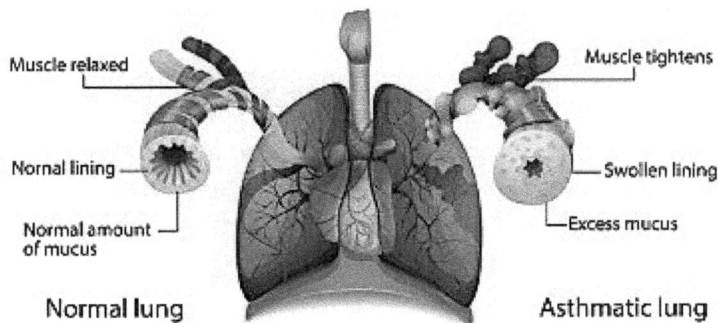

Asthma is a chronic inflammation of the airways in the lungs that can cause difficul- ty in breathing. Triggers can include allergen exercise, and respiratory infections.

Overview
To understand asthma, it helps to know how the airways work.
- The airways are tubes that carry air into and out of your lungs.
- People who have asthma have inflamed airways. The inflammation makes the airways swollen and very sensitive.
- The airways tend to react strongly to certain inhaled substances.
- When the airways react, the muscles around them tighten. This narrows the airways, causing less air to flow into the lungs.
- The swelling also can worsen, making the airways even narrower.
- Cells in the airways might make more mucus than usual. Mucus is a sticky, thick liquid that can further narrow the airways.
- This chain reaction can result in asthma symptoms. Symptoms can happen each time the airways are inflamed.

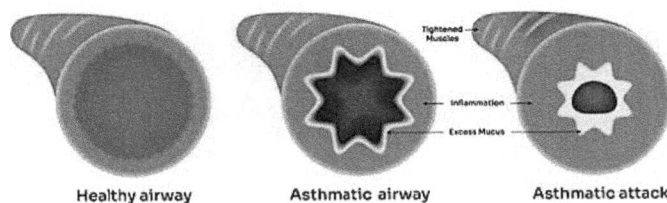

Asthma **Common Signs and Symptoms**	**Common Signs and Symptoms** <ul><li>**Coughing**. Coughing from asthma often is worse at night or early in the morning, making it hard to sleep.</li><li>**Wheezing**. Wheezing is a whistling or squeaky sound that occurs when you breathe.</li><li>**Chest tightness**. This may feel like something is squeezing or sitting on your chest.</li><li>**Shortness of breath**. Some people who have asthma say they can't catch their breath, or they feel out of breath. You may feel like you cannot get air out of your lungs.</li></ul>Not all people who have asthma have these symptoms. Likewise, having these symptoms does not always mean that you have asthma.<ul><li>The best way to diagnose asthma for certain is to use a lung function test, a medical history (including type and frequency of symptoms), and a physical exam.</li></ul>The types of asthma symptoms you have, how often they occur, and how severe they are may vary over time.<ul><li>Sometimes your symptoms may just annoy you.</li><li>Other times, they may be troublesome enough to limit your daily routine.</li><li>Severe symptoms can be fatal. It's important to treat symptoms when you first notice them so they don't become severe.</li></ul>***What Causes Asthma Symptoms To Occur?*** Many things can trigger or worsen asthma symptoms. Your doctor will help you find out which things (sometimes called triggers) may cause your asthma to flare up if you come in contact with them. **Triggers may include:**<ul><li>Allergens from dust, animal fur, cockroaches, mold, and pollens from trees, grasses, and flowers</li><li>Irritants such as cigarette smoke, air pollution, chemicals or dust in the workplace, compounds in home décor products, and sprays (such as hairspray)</li><li>Medicines such as aspirin or other nonsteroidal anti-inflammatory drugs and nonselective beta-blockers</li><li>Sulfites in foods and drinks</li><li>Viral upper respiratory infections, such as colds</li><li>Physical activity, including exercise</li><li>Other health conditions can make asthma harder to manage. Examples of these conditions include a runny nose, sinus infections, reflux disease, psychological stress, and sleep apnea. These conditions need treatment as part of an overall asthma care plan.</li></ul>

Asthma **Control and Treatment**	***Taking an active role to control your asthma involves:*** • Working with your doctor to treat other conditions that can interfere with asthma management. • Avoiding things that worsen your asthma (asthma triggers). However, one trigger you should not avoid is physical activity. Physical activity is an important part of a healthy lifestyle. Talk with your doctor about medicines that can help you stay active. Asthma is treated with two types of medicines: long-term control and quick-relief medicines. • **Long-term control** medicines help reduce airway inflammation and prevent asthma symptoms. • **Quick- relief, or "rescue,"** medicines relieve asthma symptoms that may flare up. ***Avoid Things That Can Worsen Your Asthma*** • Many common things (called asthma triggers) can set off or worsen your asthma symptoms. Once you know what these things are, you can take steps to control many of them. • For example, exposure to pollens or air pollution might make your asthma worse. If so, try to limit time outdoors when the levels of these substances in the outdoor air are high. If animal fur triggers your asthma symptoms, keep pets with fur out of your home or bedroom. • One possible asthma trigger you should not avoid is physical activity. Physical activity is an important part of a healthy lifestyle. Talk with your doctor about medicines that can help you stay active. • If your asthma symptoms are clearly related to allergens, and you cannot avoid exposure to those allergens, your doctor may advise you to get allergy shots. • You may need to see a specialist if you are thinking about getting allergy shots. These shots can lessen or prevent your asthma symptoms, but they cannot cure your asthma. • Several health conditions can make asthma harder to manage. These conditions include runny nose, sinus infections, reflux disease, psychological stress, and sleep apnea. Your doctor will treat these conditions as well. ***Watch for Signs That Your Asthma Is Getting Worse*** Your asthma might be getting worse if: • Your symptoms start to occur more often, are more severe, or bother you at night and cause you to lose sleep. • You are limiting your normal activities and missing school or work because of your asthma. • Your peak flow number is low compared to your personal best or varies a lot from day to day. • Your asthma medicines do not seem to work well anymore. • You have to use your quick-relief inhaler more often. If you are using quick-relief medicineor me than 2 days a week, your asthma is not well controlled. • You have to go to the emergency room or doctor because of an asthma attack.
Diet	**Best Foods:** Apples, Avocado, Caffeine, Cantaloupe, Carrots, Cold water fish including cod, salmon, mackerel and halibut, Extra virgin olive oil, Flax Seed, Garlic, Kale, Kiwi, Onions, Spinach, Sweet potatoes, Tomatoes **Worse Foods:** Most common for food allergies: Dairy, Eggs, Peanuts, Salt, Shellfish, Soybeans, Tree nuts, Wheat **Vitamins / Mineral**: Beta-carotene, Magnesium, Selenium, Vitamin C, Vitamin E (*Worlds Healthiest Foods*) **Supplements, Herbs, Spices or Foods containing:** Echinacea, Ginger, Glycyrrhiza (Licorice), Lobelia,Omega-3 fatty acid, Oregano, Peppermint, Quercetin, Reish mushroom, Rosemary, Sage, Turmeric **Avoid:** MSG, Omega-6 fatty acids, Salt, Tartrazine, or yellow dye #5

Asthma
 	
Medications
	Asthma medicines can be taken in pill form, but most are taken using a device called an inhaler. An inhaler allows the medicine to go directly to your lungs.
	
	Long-Term Control Medicines
	• Most people who have asthma need to take long-term control medicines daily to help prevent symptoms.
	   ▪ The most effective long-term medicines reduce airway inflammation,which helps prevent symptoms from starting. These medicines do not give you quick relief from symptoms.
	• Inhaled corticosteroids are the preferred medicine for long-term control of asthma.
	   ▪ They are the most effective option for long-term relief of the inflammation and swelling that makes your airways sensitive to certain inhaled substances.
	• Reducing inflammation helps prevent the chain reaction that causes asthma symptoms.
	   ▪ Most people who take these medicines daily find they greatly reduce the severity of symptoms and how often they occur.
	• Your doctor may prescribe low-dose inhaled corticosteroids that you will need to take each day. If your symptoms get worse, your doctor may prescribe higher doses to prevent severe flare-ups.
	   ▪ However, one study of children between the ages of 5 and 11 found that children given the higher doses when their symptoms worsened did not experience fewer severe flare-ups.
	   ▪ More frequent or prolonged high-dose inhaled corticosteroids in children in this age group may also affect growth.
	• Your doctor may have you add another long-term asthma control medicine so he or she can lower your dose of corticosteroids.
	• Inhaled corticosteroids generally are safe when taken as prescribed.
	   ▪ These medicines are different from the illegal anabolic steroids taken by some athletes.
	   ▪ Inhaled corticosteroidsare not habit-forming, even if you take them every day for many years.
	• Like many other medicines, though, inhaled corticosteroids can have side effects. Most doctors agree that the benefits of taking inhaled corticosteroids and preventing asthma attacks far outweigh the risk of side effects.
	• One common side effect from inhaled corticosteroids is a mouth infection called thrush.
	   ▪ You might be able to use a spacer or holding chamber on your inhaler to avoid thrush. These devices attach to your inhaler. They help prevent the medicine from landing in your mouth or on the back of your throat.
	• Check with your doctor to see whether a spacer or holding chamber should be used with the inhaler you have.
	   ▪ Also, work with your health care team if you have any questions about how to use a spacer or holding chamber.
	   ▪ Rinsing your mouth out with water after taking inhaled corticosteroids also can lower your risk for thrush.
	• If you have severe asthma, you may have to take corticosteroid pills or liquid for short periods to get your asthma under control.
	• If taken for long periods, these medicines raise your risk for cataracts and osteoporosis.
	   ▪ A cataract is the clouding of the lens in your eye.
	   ▪ Osteoporosis is a disorder that makes your bones weak and more likely to break. Your doctor may suggest you take calcium and vitamin D pills to protect your bones. High doses of these medicines over time may have other side effects that your doctor will monitor.

Asthma
 	
Medications
 	
Continued
	Other long-term control medicines include:
	• *Anti-inflammatory* medicine, such as cromolyn. This medicine is taken using a device calleda nebulizer. As you breathe in, the nebulizer sends a fine mist of medicine to your lungs. Cromolyn helps prevent airway inflammation.
	• *Immunomodulators,* such as omalizumab. This medicine is given as a shot (injection) one or two times a month. It helps prevent your body from reacting to asthma triggers, such as pollen and dust mites.
	  ▪ Anti-IgE might be used if other asthma medicines have not worked well. A rare, but possibly life-threatening allergic reaction called anaphylaxis might occur when the Omalizumab injection is given.
	  ▪ If you take this medication, work with your doctor to make sure you understand the signs and symptoms of anaphylaxis and what actions you should take.
	• *Inhaled long-acting beta2-agonists.* These medicines open the airways. They might be added to inhaled corticosteroids to improve asthma control. Inhaled long-acting beta 2-agonists should never be used on their own for long-term asthma control. They must be used with inhaled corticosteroids.
	• *Leukotriene* modifiers. These medicines are taken by mouth. They help block the reaction that increases inflammation in your airways.
	• *Theophylline.* This medicine is taken by mouth. Theophylline helps open the airways.
	
	If your doctor prescribes a long-term control medicine, take it every day to control your asthma.
	• Your asthma symptoms will likely return or get worse if you stop taking your medicine.
	• Long-term control medicines can have side effects. Talk with your doctor about these side effects and ways to reduce or avoid them.
	• With some medicines, like theophylline, your doctor will check the level of medicine in your blood. This helps ensure that you are getting enough medicine to relieve your asthma symptoms, but not so much that it causes dangerous side effects.
	
	Quick-Relief Medicines
	• All people who have asthma need quick-relief medicines to help relieve asthma symptoms that may flare up. Inhaled short-acting beta2-agonists are the first choice for quick relief.
	• These medicines act quickly to relax tight muscles around your airways when you are having a flareup. This allows the airways to open so air can flow through them.
	• You should take your quick-relief medicine when you first notice asthma symptoms. If you use this medicine more than 2 days a week, talk with your doctor about your asthma control. You may need to make changes to your asthma action plan.
	• Carry your quick-relief inhaler with you at all times in case you need it.
	  ▪ If your *child* has asthma, make sure that anyone caring for him or her has the child's quick-relief medicines, including staff at the child's school.
	  ▪ They should understand when and how to use these medicines and when to seek medical care for your child.
	• You should not use quick-relief medicines in place of prescribed long-term control medicines. Quick-relief medicines do not reduce inflammation.

Asthma
 	
Exercise
 	
*WebMD,
MedicineNet,*
and
*Exercise is
Medicine.org*
	What Types of Exercise Are Best for People with Asthma? *(WebMD)*
	• Activities that involve *short, intermittent periods* of exertion, such as walking, hiking, volleyball, gymnastics, baseball, and wrestling, are generally *well tolerated* by people with symptoms of asthma.
	   o Swimming, which is a strong endurance sport, is generally well tolerated by many people with asthma, because it is usually performed while breathing warm, moist air. It is also an excellent activity for maintaining physical fitness.
	• Activities that may be *less tolerated involve long periods of exertion*, such as soccer, distance running, basketball, and field hockey.
	   o Also, cold-weather sports, such as ice hockey, cross-country skiing, and ice-skating, may pose challenges.
	   o However, many people with asthma are able to participate fully in these activities.
	
	According to *MedicineNet*, it might be helpful to talk to a doctor before starting an exercise routine.
	This is especially important with asthma symptoms that worsen with exercise.
	• Many people with asthma benefit from taking a short-acting bronchodilator (such as albuterol [Ventolin, Proventil, Proventil-HFA, AccuNeb, Vospire, ProAir]) about 15 minutes before starting exercise.
	• In extremely cold or hot weather, or if there is a high level of pollution, it may best to exercise indoors. This also applies to patients with both asthma and allergies when the pollen count is high.
	
	Here are some good tips for exercising with asthma: *(Exercise is Medicine.org)*
	• Try to breathe through the nose as much as possible.
	• Wear a scarf or mask over the nose and mouth in cold weather.
	• Avoid outdoor exercise when pollen counts are high if allergies are present with asthma.
	• Avoid exercising outdoors if air pollution is high.
	• Do not exercise when sick.
	• Include a cool-down routine after exercise.
	• Do not overexert during exercise.
	• Carry an albuterol inhaler for rescue if needed.

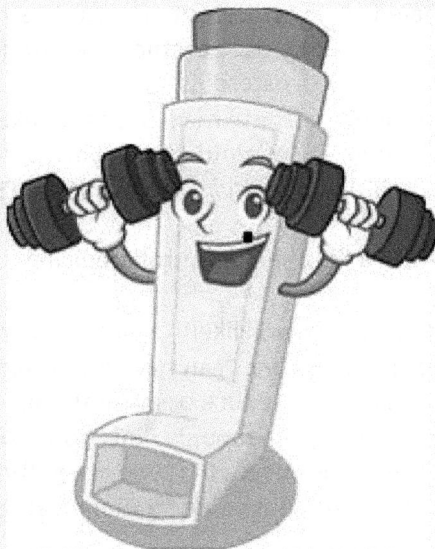

Asthma
 	
Exercise
 	
Continued
 	
Pescatello
	Aerobic Exercise Cautions
	Avoid exercising at the coldest times of the day (early morning or evening). Also,do not exercise when pollution or allergens are at their highest. Instead, exercise indoors.
	• Watch out for irritants such as smoke or allergens.
	• Warm up for 10 minutes before you exercise. This can reduce the duration and severity of an attack during and after exercise.
	• Cool down for 10 minutes after your exercise.
	• If you have been inactive for a long time, start with short sessions (10 to 15 minutes). Add five minutes to each session, increasing every two to four weeks. Gradually build up to being active at least 30 minutes a day for most days of the week.
	• Drink plenty of fluids before, during, and after exercise.
	• Do not exercise at an intensity that is too high for you. Doing so might provoke an attack and temporarily prevent exercising.
	   ▪ It also increases the risk of injury.
	
	Resistance Exercise Cautions
	• Avoid holding your breath when lifting. This can cause large changes in blood pressure.
	   ▪ That change may increase the risk of passing out or developing abnormal heart rhythms.
	• If you have joint problems or other health problems, do only one set for all major muscle groups.
	   ▪ Start with 10 to 15 repetitions. Build up to 15 to 20 repetitions before you add another set.
	
	Design your exercise program for maximum benefit and minimum risk to your health and physical condition.
	• Consider reaching out to a health and fitness EIM Professional to work with you and your doctor.
	• Together, you can establish realistic goals and design a safe, effective, and enjoyable program. *(Pescatello)*

Bronchitis

Acute Bronchitis

- Infections or lung irritants cause acute bronchitis. The same viruses that cause colds and the flu are the mostcommon cause of acute bronchitis. Sometimes bacteria can cause the condition.
- Certain substances can irritate your lungs and airways and raise your risk for acute bronchitis. For example, inhaling or being exposed to tobacco smoke, dust, fumes, vapors, or air pollution raises your risk for the condition. These lung irritants also can make symptoms worse.
- Being exposed to a high level of dust or fumes, such as from an explosion or a big fire, also may lead to acute bronchitis.

BRONCHITIS

Normal bronchial tube

Mucus

Bronchial tube with bronchitis

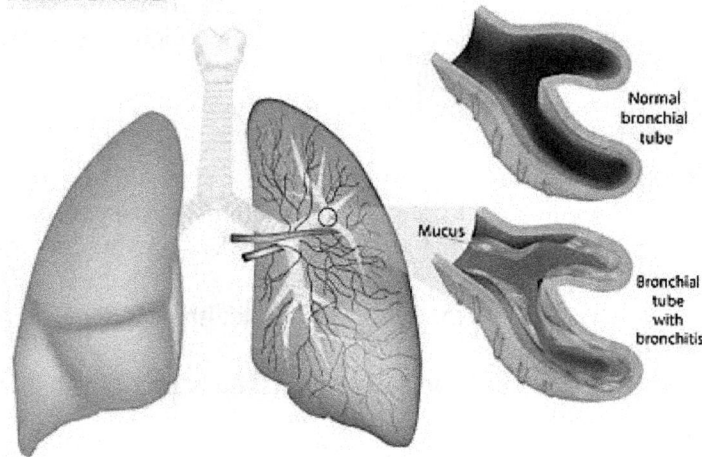

Chronic Bronchitis

- Repeatedly breathing in fumes that irritate and damage lung and airway tissues causes chronic bronchitis.Smoking is the major cause of the condition.
- Breathing in air pollution and dust or fumes from the environment or workplace also can lead to chronic bronchitis.
- People who have chronic bronchitis go through periods when symptoms become much worse than usual. During these times, they also may have acute viral or bacterial bronchitis.

Signs, Symptoms, and Complications	**Acute Bronchitis** - Acute bronchitis caused by an infection usually develops after you already have a cold orthe flu. Symptoms of a cold or the flu include sore throat, fatigue (tiredness), fever, bodyaches, stuffy or runny nose, vomiting, and diarrhea. - The main symptom of acute bronchitis is a persistent cough, which may last 10 to 20 days. The cough may produce clear mucus (a slimy substance). If the mucus is yellow or green, you may have a bacterial infection as well. Even after the infection clears up, you may still have a dry cough for days or weeks. - Other symptoms of acute bronchitis include wheezing (a whistling or squeaky sound when you breathe), low fever, and chest tightness or pain. - If your acute bronchitis is severe, you also may have shortness of breath, especially with physical activity. **Chronic Bronchitis** - The signs and symptoms of chronic bronchitis include coughing, wheezing, and chest discomfort. The coughing may produce large amounts of mucus. - This type of cough often is called a smoker's cough.

Bronchitis
 	
Treatment
	• The main goals of treating acute and chronic bronchitis are to relieve symptoms and make breathing easier.
	• If you have acute bronchitis, your doctor may recommend rest, plenty of fluids, and aspirin (for adults) or acetaminophen to treat fever.
	• Antibiotics usually are not prescribed for acute bronchitis. This is because they do not work against viruses—the most common cause of acute bronchitis.
	    o However, if your doctor thinks you have a bacterial infection, he or she may prescribe antibiotics.
	• A humidifier or steam can help loosen mucus and relieve wheezing and limited air flow. If your bronchitis causes wheezing, you may need an inhaled medicine to open your airways.
	    o You take this medicine using an inhaler.
	    o This device allows the medicine to go straight to your lungs.
	• Your doctor also may prescribe medicines to relieve or reduce your cough and treat your inflamed airways (especially if your cough persists).
	• If you have chronic bronchitis and also have been diagnosed with COPD (chronic obstructive pulmonary disease), you may need medicines to open your airways and help clear away mucus.
	    o These medicines include bronchodilators (inhaled) and steroids (inhaled or pill form).
	• If you have chronic bronchitis, your doctor may prescribe oxygen therapy.
	    o This treatment can help you breathe easier, and it provides your body with needed oxygen.

Bronchitis
 	
Exercise
 	
Medical News Today
	Acute bronchitis
	What kind and intensity of exercises are appropriate for someone with bronchitis depends on individual needs. It should be safe to exercise if cold or flu symptoms are limited to above the neck. This includes symptoms that affect:
	• Sinuses
	• Throat
	• Head
	
	Those with acute bronchitis, however, should refrain from physical exertion while they have symptoms.
	• Typically, this means avoiding purposeful exercise, during the 3–10 day recovery window.
	• Once symptoms resolve, it is usually safe to return to low levels of activity. This is the case even if a dry cough remains.
	
	Getting back to regular activity levels may take several weeks after acute bronchitis.
	• The lungs often remain inflamed after apparent recovery. This makes them less able to handle stress andmore reactive to it.
	
	Starting with more gentle exercises, or reduced versions of workouts will help the lungs slowly rebuild strength.
	• Cutting the normal duration, frequency, and intensity of workouts in half is a good starting point for many.
	
	Chronic bronchitis
	For those with chronic bronchitis, the idea of exercise may seem daunting, however, regular cardiovascular activity is key to maintaining lung health during and after episodes.
	• As with acute cases, those with chronic bronchitis should ease their way into workout routines.
	• A doctor or medical professional should be consulted to help guide the process.
	
	There are two key exercise techniques that may help:
	• **Interval exercises**: For those with chronic lung conditions, the European Lung Foundation recommend using intermittent or interval exercises, which alternate between a few minutes of activity, then rest, to help reduce shortness of breath.
	• **Controlled breathing exercises**: These include pursed lip and belly breathing. They slow exhalation, keeping the airways open longer and allowing in more air. The American Lung Association recommends doing both exercises for 5-10 minutes daily to improve symptoms, such as shortness of breath.
	   ○ *Pursed lip breathing* involves breathing in through the nose. People then slowly and steadily exhale through pursed lips for twice as long as their inhalation.
	   ○ *Belly breathing (Diaphragmatic)* requires the same inhalation and exhalation process. However, it is done without pursed lips and attention focuses on the rise and fall of the belly. It is important to keep the head, neck, and shoulders relaxed during breathing exercises. This helps ensure the diaphragm is doing the bulk of the work and retraining the way it needs.

Bronchitis **Exercise** *Continued*	***Exercises and considerations recommended for those recovering from acute bronchitis or with chronic bronchitis include:*** • Gentle stretching exercises, such as yoga, avoiding downward or upside-down poses, as these encourage phlegm to travel upwards • Cardiovascular exercises that promote light, continuous exertion, including walking or distance swimming • Continuing everyday activities or hobbies if possible or as symptoms lessen, including housework, gardening, dog walks, or playing golf • Following a steady, comfortable pace and not pushing it • Warming up and cooling down after exercise, allowing breathing rate to increase slowly and return to normal • Focusing on improving muscle strength to improve oxygen inefficiency and decrease demand on the lungs • Focusing on the duration of exertion rather than the intensity • Mindful breathing, paying attention to the length and frequency of breath • Using a humidifier before exercising to help open the airways and loosen mucus • Adjusting a workout to meet changes in weather or environmental conditions • Taking as many breaks or rest periods as needed • Drinking plenty of fluids while exercising • Keeping in mind that it may take time, from weeks to months, to see significant results and return to normal routines • Basing the intensity of workouts on what feels comfortable instead of other factors, such as heart rate or overheating • People with chronic bronchitis may find it easier to walk with their arms braced by a walker, or even by holding onto their pant waistline or belt. Some may also need to use an oxygen machine before exercise. ***Precautions When Exercising with Bronchitis*** Exercise can help lessen the symptoms of bronchitis and speed up the recovery process, by improving muscle strength and oxygen efficiency. The oxygen levels demanded by physical exertion can exceed lung capabilities, especially when airways are compromised. **Exercise should be immediately stopped if shortness of breath is intense.** • A good rule to follow is that if a person no longer has enough airflow to talk, they have gone too far. Other symptoms that indicate exercise should be stopped immediately include: • Coughing • Wheezing • Chest pain, especially a feeling similar to indigestion • Uncomfortable increase in chest tightness • Feeling faint or lightheaded • Increase in body aches or pain • Brownish, yellow-colored urine Stamina should increase over time with consistent, progressively challenging exercise. • If breathing problems continue to interfere with proper exercise, a doctor should be seen to reassess workout regimes or treatment plans.

Cystic Fibrosis

Cystic fibrosis, or CF, is an inherited disease of the secretory glands. Secretory glands include glands that make mucus and sweat. "Inherited" means the disease is passed from parents to children through genes.

- People who have CF inherit two faulty genes for the disease—one from each parent. The parents likely do not have the disease themselves.
- CF mainly affects the lungs, pancreas, liver, intestines, sinuses, and sex organs.

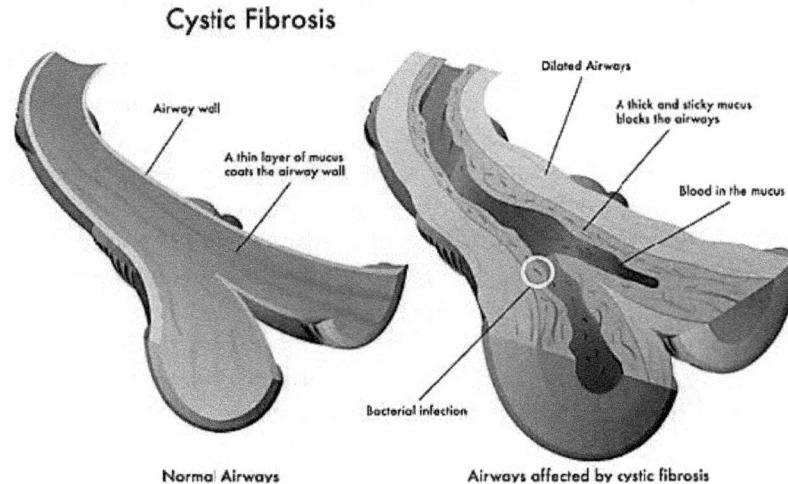

Cystic Fibrosis

Normal Airways   Airways affected by cystic fibrosis

Overview

Mucus is a substance made by tissues that line some organs and body cavities, such as the lungs and nose. Normally, mucus is a slippery, watery substance. It keeps the linings of certain organs moist and prevents them from drying out or getting infected. If you have CF, your mucus becomes thick and sticky. It builds up in your lungs and blocks your airways. (Airways are tubes that carry air in and out of your lungs.)

- The buildup of mucus makes it easy for bacteria to grow. This leads to repeated, serious lung infections. Over time, these infections can severely damage your lungs.
- The thick, sticky mucus also can block tubes, or ducts, in your pancreas (an organ in your abdomen). As a result, the digestive enzymes that your pancreas makes cannot reach your small intestine. These enzymes help break down food. Without them, your intestines cannot fully absorb fats and proteins. This can cause vitamin deficiency and malnutrition because nutrients pass through your body without being used. You also may have bulky stools, intestinal gas, a swollen belly from severe constipation, and pain or discomfort.
- CF also causes your sweat to become very salty. Thus, when you sweat, you lose large amounts of salt. This can upset the balance of minerals in your blood and cause many health problems. Examples of these problems include dehydration (a lack of fluid in your body), increased heart rate, fatigue (tiredness), weakness, decreased blood pressure, heat stroke, and, rarely, death.
- If you or your child has CF, you are also at higher risk for diabetes, or two bone-thinning conditions called osteoporosis and osteopenia.
- CF also causes infertility in men, and the disease can make it harder for women to get pregnant. (The term"infertility" refers to the inability to have children.)

Outlook

- The symptoms and severity of CF vary. If you or your child has the disease, you may have serious lung and digestive problems. If the disease is mild, symptoms may not show up until the teen or adult years.
- The symptoms and severity of CF also vary over time. Sometimes you will have few symptoms. Other times,your symptoms may become more severe. As the disease gets worse, you will have more severe symptoms more often.
- Lung function often starts to decline in early childhood in people who have CF. Over time, damage to the lungs can cause severe breathing problems. Respiratory failure is the most common cause of death in people who have CF.

Cystic fibrosis Signs, Symptoms, and Complications	The signs and symptoms of cystic fibrosis (CF) vary from person to person and over time. Sometimes you will have few symptoms. Other times, your symptoms may become more severe. • One of the first signs of CF that parents may notice is that their baby's skin tastes salty when kissed, or the baby does not pass stool when first born. • Most of the other signs and symptoms of CF happen later. They are related to how CF affects the respiratory, digestive, or reproductive systems of the body. ***Respiratory System Signs and Symptoms*** • Thick, sticky mucus that builds up in their airways. This buildup of mucus makes it easier for bacteria to grow and cause infections. Infections can block the airways and cause frequent coughing that brings up thick sputum (spit) or mucus that is sometimes bloody. • Tend to have lung infections caused by unusual germs that do not respond to standard antibiotics. For example, lung infections caused by bacteria called mucoid Pseudomonas are much more common in people who have CF than in those who do not. An infection caused by these bacteria may be a sign of CF. • Frequent bouts of sinusitis, an infection of the sinuses. The sinuses are hollow air spaces around the eyes, nose, and forehead. Frequent bouts of bronchitis and pneumonia also can occur. These infections can cause long-term lung damage. • As CF gets worse, you may have more serious problems, such as pneumothorax or bronchiectasis. • Some people who have CF also develop nasal polyps (growths in the nose) that may require surgery. ***Digestive System Signs and Symptoms*** In CF, mucus can block tubes, or ducts, in your pancreas (an organ in your abdomen). These blockages prevent enzymes from reaching your intestines. As a result, your intestines cannot fully absorb fats and proteins. • This can cause ongoing diarrhea or bulky, foul-smelling, greasy stools. Intestinal blockages also may occur, especially in newborns. Too much gas or severe constipation in the intestines may cause stomach pain and discomfort. ***As CF gets worse, other problems may occur, such as***: • Pancreatitis. This is a condition in which the pancreas become inflamed, which causes pain. • Rectal prolapse. Frequent coughing or problems passing stools may cause rectal tissue from inside you to move out of your rectum. • Liver disease due to inflamed or blocked bile ducts. • Diabetes. • Gallstones. ***Reproductive System Signs and Symptoms*** • Men who have CF are infertile because they are born without a vas deferens. The vas deferens is a tube that delivers sperm from the testes to the penis. • Women who have CF may have a hard time getting pregnant because of mucus blocking the cervix or other CF complications. ***Other Signs, Symptoms, and Complications*** Other signs and symptoms of CF are related to an upset of the balance of minerals in your blood. • CF causes your sweat to become very salty. As a result, your body loses large amounts of salt when you sweat. This can cause dehydration (a lack of fluid in your body), increased heart rate, fatigue (tiredness), weakness, decreased blood pressure, heat stroke, and, rarely, death. • CF also can cause clubbing and low bone density. Clubbing is the widening and rounding of the tips of your fingers and toes. This sign develops late in CF because your lungs are not moving enough oxygen into your bloodstream. • Low bone density also tends to occur late in CF. It can lead to bone-thinning disorders called osteoporosis and osteopenia.

Cystic fibrosis
 	
Treatment
	Treatment for Lung Problems
	
	Exercise *(Also see Below)*
	• Aerobic exercise that makes you breathe harder can help loosen the mucus in your airways so you can cough it up. Exercise also helps improve your overall physical condition.
	• However, CF causes your sweat to become very salty. As a result, your body loses large amounts of salt when you sweat. Thus, your doctor may recommend a high-salt diet or salt supplements to maintain the balance of minerals in your blood.
	• If you exercise regularly, you may be able to cut back on your CPT (chest physical therapy), however, you should check with your doctor first.
	
	Chest Physical Therapy (CPT)
	• CPT also is called chest clapping or percussion. It involves pounding your chest and back over and over with your hands or a device to loosen the mucus from your lungs so that you can cough it up.
	• You might sit down or lie on your stomach with your head down while you do CPT. Gravityand force help drain the mucus from your lungs.
	• Some people find CPT hard or uncomfortable to do.
	Several devices have been developed that may help with CPT, such as:
	    o An electric chest clapper, known as a mechanical percussor.
	    o An inflatable therapy vest that uses high-frequency airwaves to force the mucus that is deep in your lungs toward your upper airways so you can cough it up.
	    o A small, handheld device that you exhale through. The device causes vibrations that dislodge the mucus.
	    o A mask that creates vibrations that help break the mucus loose from your airway walls.
	    o Breathing techniques also may help dislodge mucus so you can cough it up. These techniques include forcing out a couple of short breaths or deeper breaths and then doing relaxed breathing. This may help loosen the mucus in your lungs and open your airways.
	
	Medicines
	If you have CF, your doctor may prescribe antibiotics, anti-inflammatory medicines, bronchodilators, or medicines to help clear the mucus. These medicines help treat or prevent lung infections, reduce swelling, open up the airways, and thin mucus. If you have mutations in a gene called G551D, which occurs in about 5 percent of people who have CF, your doctor may prescribe the oral medicine ivacaftor (approved for people with CF who are 6 years of age and older).
	• Antibiotics are the main treatment to prevent or treat lung infections. Your doctor may prescribe oral, inhaled, or intravenous (IV) antibiotics.
	• Oral antibiotics often are used to treat mild lung infections.
	• Inhaled antibiotics may be used to prevent or control infections caused by the bacteria mucoid Pseudomonas.
	• For severe or hard-to-treat infections, you may be given antibiotics through an IV tube (a tube inserted into a vein). This type of treatment may require you to stay in a hospital.
	• Anti-inflammatory medicines can help reduce swelling in your airways due to ongoing infections. These medicines may be inhaled or oral.
	• Bronchodilators help open the airways by relaxing the muscles around them. These medicines are inhaled. They are often taken just before CPT to help clear mucus out of your airways. You also may take bronchodilators before inhaling other medicines into your lungs.
	• Your doctor may prescribe medicines to reduce the stickiness of your mucus and loosen it up. These medicines can help clear out mucus, improve lung function, and prevent worsening lung symptoms.

Cystic fibrosis **Treatment** *Continued*	**Treatments for Advanced Lung Disease** If you have advanced lung disease, you may need oxygen therapy. Oxygen usually is given through nasal prongs or a mask. • If other treatments have not worked, a lung transplant may be an option if you have severe lung disease. A lung transplant is surgery to remove a person's diseased lung and replace it with a healthy lung from a deceased donor.

Pulmonary Rehabilitation (PR)

Your doctor may recommend PR as part of your treatment plan. PR is a broad program that helps improve the well-being of people who have chronic (ongoing) breathing problems. PR does not replace medical therapy. Instead, it is used with medical therapy and may include:

- Exercise training
- Nutritional counseling
- Education on your lung disease or condition and how to manage it
- Energy-conserving techniques
- Breathing strategies
- Psychological counseling and/or group support
- PR has many benefits. It can improve your ability to function and your quality of life. The program also may help relieve your breathing problems. Even if you have advanced lung disease, you can still benefit from PR.

Treatment for Digestive Problems

CF can cause many digestive problems, such as bulky stools, intestinal gas, a swollen belly, severe constipation, and pain or discomfort.

- Digestive problems also can lead to poor growth and development in children.
- Nutritional therapy can improve your strength and ability to stay active. It also can improve growthand development in children.
- Nutritional therapy also may make you strong enough to resist somelung infections. A nutritionist can help you create a nutritional plan that meets your needs.

In addition to having a well-balanced diet that is rich in calories, fat, and protein, your nutritional therapy may include:

- Oral pancreatic enzymes to help you digest fats and proteins and absorb more vitamins.
- Supplements of vitamins A, D, E, and K to replace the fat-soluble vitamins that your intestines cannot absorb.
- High calorie shakes to provide you with extra nutrients.
- A high-salt diet or salt supplements that you take before exercising.
- A feeding tube to give you more calories at night while you are sleeping. The tube may be threaded through your nose and throat and into your stomach or the tube may be placed directly into your stomach through a surgically made hole.
  - Before you go to bed each night,you will attach a bag with a nutritional solution to the entrance of the tube. It will feed you while you sleep.
- Other treatments for digestive problems may include enemas and mucus-thinning medicines to treat intestinal blockages.
- Sometimes surgery is needed to remove anintestinal blockage.
- Your doctor also may prescribe medicines to reduce your stomach acid and help oral pancreatic enzymes work better.

Treatments for Cystic Fibrosis Complications

- A common complication of CF is diabetes. The type of diabetes associated with CF often requires different treatment than other types of diabetes.
- Another common CF complication is the bone-thinning disorder osteoporosis. Your doctor may prescribe medicines that prevent your bones from losing their density.

Cystic fibrosis **Exercise** *MedScape*	Research studies have shown that individuals with cystic fibrosis who attain higher levels of aerobic fitness report feeling better and having a higher overall quality of life. <ul><li>And, while cystic fibrosis can certainly make exercise more challenging, regular physical activity may actually improve your symptoms, particularly mucus clearance, and possibly even delay decreases in your pulmonary function.</li><li>Start exercising regularly and you will likely find it much easier to perform everyday tasks as well.</li><li>The key is to determine what type of exercise is best for you and to follow a program that accommodates your individual needs and concerns.</li></ul>

ORGANS AFFECTED BY CYSTIC FIBROSIS

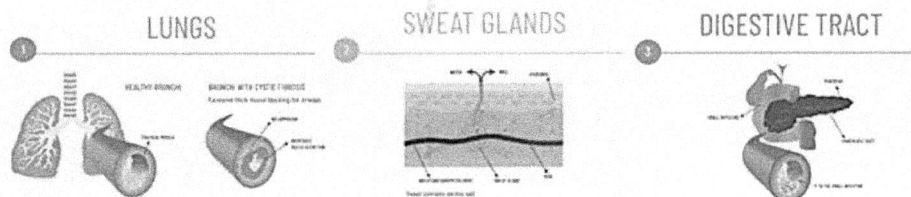

LUNGS   SWEAT GLANDS   DIGESTIVE TRACT

Talk with your health care provider before starting an exercise program and ask for specific programming recommendations.

Getting Started

- Take all medications as recommended by your physician.
- The goals of your program should be to increase your cardiovascular fitness, facilitate mucus clearance, and improve your ability to perform activities of daily living.
- Choose activities that you enjoy such as walking, cycling, rowing, and swimming and work up to a moderate intensity.
- Start slowly and gradually increase the intensity and duration of your workouts. You may need to start with 5 - to 10-minute sessions and build up to 30-minute sessions, three or more days per week.
- Two days per week do three 10-repetition sets of light-resistance strength-training exercises targeting all the major muscle groups. Use the Ratings of Perceived Exertion and dyspnea scales as well as heart rate to measure your intensity and adjust your workouts according to fluctuations in your symptoms.

Exercise Cautions

- Supplemental oxygen may enhance your training effect. Initially, you may want to have your oxyhemoglobin saturation monitored to determine your optimal level of oxygen supplementation.
- Avoid extreme weather conditions; prolonged exercise in the heat may increase your need for fluids and dietary salt.

Your exercise program should be designed to maximize the benefits with the fewest risks of aggravating your health or physical condition.

Consider contacting a certified health and fitness professional who can work with you and your health care provider to establish realistic goals and design a safe and effective program that addresses your specific needs.

Idiopathic Pulmonary Fibrosis

Pulmonary fibrosis is a disease in which tissue deep in your lungs becomes thick and stiff, or scarred, over time. The formation of scar tissue is called fibrosis.

- As the lung tissue thickens, your lungs cannot properly move oxygen into your bloodstream. As a result, your brain and other organs do not get the oxygen they need.
- Sometimes doctors can find out what is causing fibrosis, but in most cases, they cannot find a cause. They call these cases idiopathic pulmonary fibrosis (IPF).

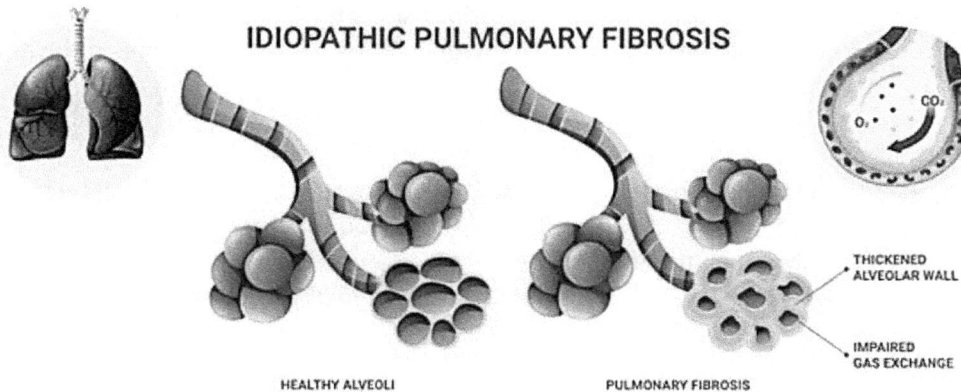

IPF is a serious disease that usually affects middle-aged and older adults.

- IPF varies from person to person. In some people, fibrosis happens quickly. In others, the process is much slower. In some people, the disease stays the same for years.
- IPF has no cure yet. Many people live only about 3 to 5 years after diagnosis. The most common cause of death related to IPF is respiratory failure. Other causes of death include pulmonary hypertension, heart failure, pulmonary embolism, pneumonia, and lung cancer.
- Genetics may play a role in causing IPF. If more than one member of your family has IPF, the disease is called familial IPF.

Signs, Symptoms, and Complications	The signs and symptoms of idiopathic pulmonary fibrosis (IPF) develop over time. They may not even begin to appear until the disease has done serious damage to your lungs. Once they occur, they are likely to get worse over time.
	The most common signs and symptoms are:
	• Shortness of breath. This usually is the main symptom of IPF. At first, you may be short of breath only during exercise. Over time, you will likely feel breathless even at rest.
	• A dry, hacking cough that does not get better. Over time, you may have repeated bouts of coughing that you cannot control.
	Other signs and symptoms that you may develop over time include:
	• Rapid, shallow breathing
	• Gradual, unintended weight loss
	• Fatigue (tiredness) or malaise (a general feeling of being unwell)
	• Aching muscles and joints
	• Clubbing, which is the widening and rounding of the tips of the fingers or toes.
	• IPF may lead to other medical problems, including a collapsed lung, lung infections, blood clots in the lungs, and lung cancer.
	• As the disease worsens, you may develop other potentially life-threatening conditions, including respiratory failure, pulmonary hypertension, and heart failure.

Pulmonary fibrosis **Treatment**	*Medicines* Currently, no medicines are proven to slow the progression of IPF. Prednisone, azathioprine, and N-acetylcysteine have been used to treat IPF, either alone or in combination. However, experts have not found enough evidence to support their use. **Prednisone** • Prednisone is an anti-inflammatory medicine. You usually take it by mouth every day. However, your doctor may give it to you through a needle or tube inserted into a vein in your arm for several days. After that, you usually take it by mouth. • Because prednisone can cause serious side effects, your doctor may prescribe it for 3 to 6 months or less at first. Then, if it works for you, your doctor may reduce the dose over time and keep you on it longer. **Azathioprine** • Azathioprine suppresses your immune system. You usually take it by mouth every day. Because it can cause serious side effects, your doctor may prescribe it with prednisone for only 3 to 6 months. • If you do not have serious side effects and the medicines seem to help you, your doctor may keep you on them longer. **N-acetylcysteine** • N-acetylcysteine is an antioxidant that may help prevent lung damage. You usually take it by mouth several times a day. A common treatment for IPF is a combination of prednisone, azathioprine, and N- acetylcysteine. • However, this treatment was recently found harmful in a study funded by the National Heart, Lung, and Blood Institute (NHLBI). • If you have IPF and take this combination of medicines, talk with your doctor. • Do not stop taking the medicines on your own. *Other Treatments* Other treatments that may help people who have IPF include the following: • Flu and pneumonia vaccines may help prevent infections and keep you healthy. • Cough medicines or oral codeine may relieve coughing. • Vitamin D, calcium, and a bone-building medicine may help prevent bone loss if you are taking prednisone or another corticosteroid. • Anti-reflux therapy may help control gastroesophageal reflux disease (GERD). Most people who have IPF also have GERD. • Oxygen Therapy • Pulmonary Rehabilitation - PR is now a standard treatment for people who have chronic (ongoing) lung disease. PR is a broad program that helps improve the well-being of people who have breathing problems. *Lung Transplant* • Your doctor may recommend a lung transplant if your condition is quickly worsening or very severe. A lung transplant can improve your quality of life and help you live longer. • Some medical centers will consider patients older than 65 for lung transplants if they have no other serious medical problems. • The major complications of a lung transplant are rejection and infection. ("Rejection" refers to your body creating proteins that attack the new organ.) You will have to take medicines for the rest of your life to reduce the risk of rejection.

Pulmonary fibrosis **Lifestyle Changes**	No cure is available for idiopathic pulmonary fibrosis (IPF) yet. Your symptoms may get worse over time. As your symptoms worsen, you may not be able to do many of the things that you did before you had IPF, however, lifestyle changes and ongoing care can help you manage the disease. <ul><li>If you are still smoking, the most important thing you can do is quit. Talk with your doctor about programs and products that can help you quit. Also, try to avoid secondhand smoke. Ask family members and friends not to smoke in front of you or in your home, car, or workplace.</li><li>Staying active can help with both your physical and mental health. Physical activity can help you maintain your strength and lung function and reduce stress. Try moderate exercise, such as walking or riding a stationary bike. Ask your doctor about using oxygen while exercising.</li><li>As your condition advances, use a wheelchair or motorized scooter, or stay busy with activities that are not physical in nature.</li><li>You also should follow a healthy diet.<ul><li>A healthy diet includes a variety of fruits and vegetables.</li><li>It also includes whole grains, fat-free or low-fat dairy products, and protein foods, such as lean meats, poultry without skin, seafood, processed soy products, nuts, seeds, beans, and peas.</li><li>A healthy diet is low in sodium (salt), added sugars, solid fats, and refined grains. Solid fats are saturated fat and trans fatty acids.</li><li>Refined grains come from processing whole grains, which results in a loss of nutrients (such as dietary fiber).</li></ul></li><li>Eating smaller, more frequent meals may relieve stomach fullness, which can make it hard to breathe. If you need help with your diet, ask your doctor to arrange for a dietitian to work with you.</li><li>Getting plenty of rest can increase your energy and help you deal with the stress of living with a serious condition like IPF.</li><li>Try to maintain a positive attitude; relaxation techniques may help you do this. These techniques also may help you avoid excessive oxygen intake caused by tension or overworked muscles.</li><li>Avoid situations that can make your symptoms worse.<ul><li>For example, avoid traveling by air or living at or traveling to high altitudes where the air is thin and the amount of oxygen in the air is low.</li></ul></li></ul>

Pulmonary fibrosis **Exercise and Breathing Exercises** *Lung Institute*	Supervised exercise training programs have demonstrated clinical benefits in improving exercise capacity, dyspnea (difficulty breathing) and quality of life in patients with PF. • The underlying mechanisms of chronic adaption to a regular exercise regimen in PF have yet to be well- described and require further investigation. • The benefit of exercise training is well-established for chronic conditions such as pulmonary fibrosis. • Moderate levels of exercise that do not result in significantly worsened symptoms are generally safe, though it is imperative to monitor oxygen levels and be sure that the person exercising has safe blood-oxygen levels. **Pulmonary Fibrosis and Exercise** Under the *supervision of a pulmonologist*, patients with pulmonary fibrosis should exercise. • With exercise, the lungs will work at maximum efficiency, and exercise enables the heart and other muscles to do more with the oxygen available to them. • Many people find participating in pulmonary rehabilitation helpful as well. Once they learn how to exercise properly and safely, they feel ready to try exercising on their own. • In combination with exercise, staying on top of your pulmonary fibrosis treatments is important. ## Breathing Exercises ***It is important to discuss these pulmonary fibrosis breathing exercises with your doctor before trying them.*** ***Done properly, pulmonary fibrosis breathing exercises may help you breathe deeper and staycalmer.*** **Belly Breathing Technique** Belly breathing or diaphragmatic breathing helps people strengthen their diaphragm, so they breathe better. In fact, belly breathing can also be used to help people relax. This pulmonary fibrosis breathing exercise can be done while lying down or sitting in a chair. • Lie on your back with your knees bent with a pillow underneath them or sit in a comfortable chair. • Place one hand on your upper chest and the other on your belly just below your ribcage. • Inhale slowly and gently through your nose and keep the hand on your chest as still as possible. • Focus on feeling your belly move as you breathe. • Exhale slowly and gently through your mouth, keeping the hand on your chest still. • You can practice belly breathing 3-4 times a day for about 5-10 minutes.

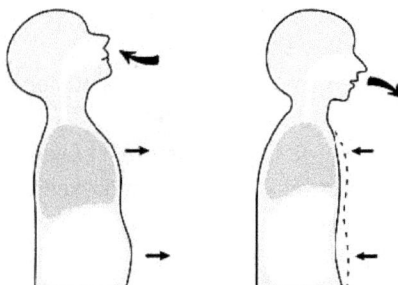

Pulmonary fibrosis **Exercise and Breathing Exercises** *Continued*	### Huff-Cough Technique Coughing is a common problem for people with pulmonary fibrosis and other chronic lung diseases as it can cause fatigue. Doctors recommend the Huff-Cough Technique to help their patients cough more effectively, so their patients do not become overly fatigued. • Sit in a comfortable chair. • Take several deep, gentle breaths as best you can, like you would in belly breathing. • Put one hand on your stomach and breathe normally. • Tighten your stomach and chest muscles. • Keep your mouth open. • Whisper the word "huff" while forcing the air out. ### Forced Coughing Technique The forced coughing technique helps remove excess mucus from your airways. Excessive mucusis a common problem for people with chronic lung diseases. Here is how to do the forced coughing technique: • Sit in a comfortable chair. • Keep your back straight and your feet pressed against the floor. • Breathe as deeply as you can. • Focus on feeling your diaphragm expand. • Hold your breath for three counts. • Open your mouth and cough twice. • If mucus comes up, discard it in a tissue. • Repeat until your airways feel clear of mucus. ### Pursed Lips Breathing Pursed lips breathing helps address shortness of breath and offers many benefits. The benefits of pursed lips breathing include opening the airways to ease breathing, relieving shortness of breath, and promoting relaxation. This technique can be done sitting, standing, or lying down. However, to maximize the benefits, many people choose to sit or lie down. • Relax your neck and shoulders. • Breathe in slowly through your nose for two seconds with your mouth closed. • Breath out slowly through your mouth for four seconds with your lips puckered. • As you exhale, keep it slow and steady. • Repeat and extend the counts as you go.

Oxygen Therapy

Oxygen therapy is a treatment that provides you with extra oxygen. Oxygen is a gas that your body needs to function. Normally, your lungs absorb oxygen from the air you breathe. But some conditions can prevent you from getting enough oxygen

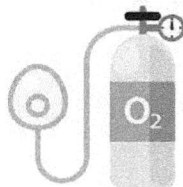

You may need oxygen if you have:
- COPD (chronic obstructive pulmonary disease)
- Pneumonia
- A severe asthma attack
- Late-stage heart failure
- Cystic fibrosis
- Sleep apnea

You can receive oxygen therapy from tubes resting in your nose, a face mask, or a tube placed in your trachea, or windpipe.
- This treatment increases the amount of oxygen your lungs receive and deliver to your blood.
- Oxygen therapy may be prescribed for you when you have a condition that causes your blood oxygen levels to be too low.
  - Low blood oxygen may make you feel short of breath, tired, or confused, and can damage your body.

Oxygen therapy can be given for a short or long period of time in the hospital, another medical setting, or at home.
- Oxygen is stored as a gas or liquid in special tanks. These tanks can be delivered to your home and contain a certain amount of oxygen that will require refills.
- Another device for use at home is an *oxygen concentrator*, which pulls oxygen out of the air for immediate use. Because oxygen concentrators do not require refills, they will not run out of oxygen.
- *Portable tanks* and oxygen concentrators may make it easier for you to move around while using your therapy.
- Oxygen poses a fire risk, so you should never smoke or use flammable materials when using oxygen.
- You may experience side effects from this treatment, such as a dry or bloody nose, tiredness, and morning headaches.
- Oxygen therapy is generally safe.
- A different kind of oxygen therapy is called *hyperbaric oxygen therapy*. It uses oxygen at high pressure to treat wounds and serious infections.

  (MedLine Plus and NIH – Oxygen)

Should I Use My Oxygen When I Exercise? *(American Lung Association)*
If you use oxygen, you should exercise with it. Your doctor may adjust your flow rate for physical activity, which will be different than your flow rate when you are resting. Work with your doctor to adjust your oxygen for physical activity.
- Here are some other tips for breathing during exercise:
- Remember to inhale (breathe in) before starting the exercise and exhale (breathe out) through the most difficult part of the exercise.
- Take slow breaths and pace yourself.
- Purse your lips while breathing out.

Respiratory References

NIH - National Heart, Lung and Blood Institute

Asthma https://www.nhlbi.nih.gov/health-topics/asthma
Bronchitis https://www.nhlbi.nih.gov/health-topics/bronchitis
COPD https://www.nhlbi.nih.gov/health- topics/copd
Cystic Fibrosis https://www.nhlbi.nih.gov/health-topics/cystic-fibrosis
Idiopathic Pulmonary Fibrosis https://www.nhlbi.nih.gov/health-topics/idiopathic-pulmonary-fibrosis
Oxygen   https://www.nhlbi.nih.gov/health-topics/oxygen-therapy

American Lung Association: *Physical Activity and COPD* http://www.lung.org/lung-health-and-diseases/lung-disease-lookup/copd/living-with-copd/physical-activity.html

COPD Store - *Signs You Should Stop Exercising*
 http://blog.copdstore.com/the-official-guide-to-exercising-with-copd

Exercise is Medicine.org - *Exercising with Asthma*
http://exerciseismedicine.org/assets/page_documents/EIM%20Rx%20series_Asthma.pdf

HealthLine: *COPD and Exercise: Tips for Breathing Better*
https://www.healthline.com/health/copd/and-exercise#1

Lung Institute - *Best Pulmonary Fibrosis Breathing Exercises*
https://lunginstitute.com/blog/best-pulmonary-fibrosis-breathing-exercises/

Lung Institute - *Can You Exercise Safely with Pulmonary Fibrosis?*
https://lunginstitute.com/blog/pulmonary-fibrosis-and-exercise/

MedScape - *Exercising With Cystic Fibrosis: Prescription for Health*
https://www.medscape.com/viewarticle/719536

Medical News Today - *Is it safe to exercise with bronchitis?*
https://www.medicalnewstoday.com/articles/317849.php

MedicineNet – *Asthma*
https://www.medicinenet.com/best_exercises_for_asthma_yoga_swimming_biking/views.htm

MedLine Plus – *Oxygen* - https://medlineplus.gov/oxygentherapy.html

Pescatello, L., Arena, R., Riebe, D., & Thompson, P. (2013). "General Principles of Exercise Prescription". *ACSM's Guidelines for Exercise Testing and Prescription* (9th ed., pp. 166-177). Philadelphia: Wolters Kluwer Health/Lippincott Williams

WebMD – *Exercise and Asthma* https://www.webmd.com/asthma/guide/exercising-asthma#1

Worlds Healthiest Foods – *Food Sensitivities* http://www.whfoods.com/genpage.php?tname=faq&dbid=30

Quick Summary this Section

Safety First
- Benefits / Before Starting a Routine
- Averages, Body Temperature
- Respiration, Blood Pressure, Heart Rate
- How to Monitor Intensity of Heart Rate
- Temperature – Heat and Cold
- Dehydration; Altitude

Components of a Conditioning Program
- Warm up/cool down
- Duration, Frequency, Intensity & Movement Patterns
- Breathing – Diaphragmatic, Pursed lip and with Exercise
- Equipment That May be Needed

Self-Tests:
- Prior to starting program

Exercise Worksheets:
- Exercises below with:
  - Exercise name and number for section
    - Reps, Sets, How many times a day and how long a stretch should be held (Ex. 20 seconds)

EXERCISE Flexibility (Stretching)	EXERCISE NUMBER	PAGE	REPS	SETS	X DAY	HOLD
PRAYER STRETCH and LATERAL	53					

Exercises:
- Myofascial release
- Flexibility / Stretches / ROM
- Core / Abdominal
- Strengthening - Upper and Lower Extremity
- Balance > Lower Extremity Standing Exercises
- Agility
- Endurance/Aerobic Capacity
- Calories
- Worksheet with room for notes under each section

EXERCISE Core / Stability / Balance	EXERCISE NUMBER	NOTES
PRONE BALL	27	

References

PHYSICAL AND PSYCHOLOGICAL BENEFITS OF KEEPING PHYSICALLY FIT

- Contributes positively to maintaining a healthy weight, building and maintaining healthy bone density, muscle strength, joint mobility, reducing surgical risks, and strengthening the immune system.
- Helps to prevent or treat serious and life-threatening chronic conditions such as high blood pressure, obesity, heart disease, Type 2 diabetes, insomnia, and depression.
- Endurance exercise before meals lowers blood glucose more than the same exercise after meals.
- It also improves mental health, helps prevent depression, helps to promote or maintain positive self-esteem, and can even augment an individual's sex appeal or body image.

(*Physical Exercise - Wikipedia*)

Before starting a routine here are some factors to consider

AGE	Men over 45 and women over 55 should have medical evaluation before starting a vigorous exercise program. If you will be participating in low to moderate exercise, it is suggested that those with, or have signs and symptoms of cardiopulmonary disease, set up a medical evaluation.
MEDICAL AND PHYSICAL CONDITION	It is very important for you to be aware of any medical or physical problems that may impede your performance. **If you have any of the following issues, please see a medical doctor and/or physical therapist to address issues before starting an exercise program:** • Cardiac issues • Pulmonary issues • Arthritis • Joint pain • Back pain • Diabetes • Acute or Chronic issues, such as, but not limited to, Parkinson's, Stroke, Autoimmune Diseases, Metabolic Disease or Orthopedic disorders/joint replacements.

VITAL SIGN AVERAGES

Adult (resting)

Body Temperature	98.6 Fahrenheit under tongue.
Respiration	12-20 breaths per minute

Blood Pressure
 	
Systolic/Diastolic
	120/80.
	Systolic is when the heart pumps blood to the body / Diastolic is blood that remains in arteries when the heart relaxes.
	Pre-hypertension: 120-139/80-89.
	Hypertension:
	    Stage I 140-159/90-99
	    Stage II over 160/100

Resting pulse	**Men:** 70 beats per minute. **Women:** 75 beats per minute.

HOW to MONITOR EXERCISE INTENSITY

Ways to monitor heart rate (HR):

Talk Test Method	This is a simple, subjective method for the beginner to determine your comfort zone while exercising. Are you able to breathe and talk comfortably throughout the workout without gasping for air? If not, reduce your activity level, catch your breath, and resume at a slower pace.
Heart Rate monitor or Watch	This is a device you wear on your wrist or chest, which allows you to measure your heart rate in real time. These devices range in price at about $50.00 for just a basic HR monitor or higher with other bells and whistles. Some of the popular manufacturers are Fitbit, Apple Watch, Garmin and Samsung Galaxy among others. (See *Target Heart Rate*)
Rate of Perceived Exertion	This method was designed by Dr. Gunnar Borg and is often called the Borg Scale (revised). It rates what you feel your level of exertion is from a scale of 1-10, one being at rest and ten at maximal exertion. A rate of 5-7 is recommended, somewhere between somewhat hard and very hard. Like the talk test method, this is subjective and should be used with HR monitoring.
Training Heart Rate	Measuring Heart Rate: Place your first and second finger over the pulse site and gently apply pressure. Palpate the number of beats for a full minute or 30 sec x 2, 15 sec x 4 or 6 sec x 10. If you have in irregular heartbeat, it is suggested counting the full 60 seconds. Do not use the thumb, as this has its own pulse.
	Take your pulse after you've been exercising for at least five minutes. An easy way to check your pulse without interrupting your workout too much is to take a quick 6-second count and then multiply that number by 10 to get your heart rate in beats per minute (BPM). Make sure your pulse is within your target heart rate zone (*see below*). You can then increase or decrease your intensity based on your heart rate. You can also wear a heart rate monitor.

Radial: Wrist following line from base of thumb.

Carotid: Side of larynx.

Target heart rate range (THR)	**Beginner or low fitness level**: 50-60%
	Intermediate or average fitness level: 60-70%
	Advanced or high fitness level: 75-85%
Percent of maximal heart rate	220 - Age = predicted maximum heart rate (HR). To get the desired exercise intensity, multiply the predicted maximal HR by the percentage. For example, a woman who is 40 years old of Intermediate fitness level would use the following equation at a 70% target heart rate: 220 – 40 (age) =180 predicted maximal HR. 180 x 0.70 (THR) = 126 BPM - desired exercise HR.
Karvonen Formula	Percentage of Heart-rate reserve. This formula factors in the resting HR as well, which will make the target heart rate higher than just the percentage of maximal heart rate. To figure this out, take the predicted maximal heart rate as above with a resting HR prior to exercise. Maximal HR – resting heart rate (RHR) = heart rate reserve; multiply by intensity + RHR + Target HR. See example under Percentage of maximal HR. Rest heart rate = 80. 220 – 40 (age) =180 (as above) – 80 (RHR) = 100 x 0.70 (THR) = 70 + 80 = 150 Target HR.

TEMPERATURE – HEAT and COLD

HEAT

Avoid exercise in the hottest part of the day, as well as in humid weather. People need to sweat to regulate internal body temperature and must evaporate to dissipate heat. During hot, humid weather, sweat cannot evaporate, and therefore cannot cool the body down. It is also important to drink plenty of cool water during exercise, about 7-10 oz. every 10-20 minutes during exercise (see *Dehydration*).

Heat cramps:	• Severe cramps that begin in hands, feet or calves • Hard, tense muscles
Heat exhaustion: Requires immediate medical attention, although not usually life threatening	• Fatigue • Nausea • Headache • Excessive thirst • Muscle aches and cramps • Confusion or anxiety • Weakness • Severe sweats that can be accompanied by cold, clammy skin • Slow heartbeat (decreased pulse rate) • Dizziness or fainting • Agitation
Heat Stroke: Can occur suddenly, with or without warning from heat exhaustion. Obtain immediate medical attention, as this can be *fatal*	• Nausea and vomiting • Headache • Increased body temperature, but DECREASED sweating. • Hot, flushed, DRY skin • Dizziness • Fatigue • Rapid heart rate • Shortness of breath • Decreased urination or may have blood in the urine. • Confusion or loss of consciousness • Convulsions

COLD

It is just as important to drink plenty of water when exercising in the cold weather secondary to increased urine production.   Be sure to dress in layers to help self-regulate body temperature. This simply involves taking off or putting back on clothing as dictated by the changing weather conditions. Choose clothing that will keep moisture out and away from the skin, such as Gortex® brand. Clothing that stays wet because of sweat will decrease your body temperature.

Hypothermia-Mild: A body temperature that is below normal. People with hypothermia are usually not aware of their condition due to confusion or being overly focused on their current activity. Hypothermia may or may not include shivering in the early stages	• Confusion • Lack of coordination • Fatigue • Nausea or vomiting • Dizziness
Hypothermia	• Shivering • Slurred speech • Mumbling • Clumsiness • Difficulty speaking • Stumbling • Poor decision making • Drowsiness • Weak pulse • Shallow breathing • Progressive loss of consciousness

DEHYDRATION

Excessive loss of body fluid (which can include water and solutes, usually sodium or electrolytes). It is also important to drink plenty of cool water during exercise, about 7-10 oz. every 10-20 minutes during exercise. During exercise, sports drinks may be necessary to keep an electrolyte balance as well.

Dehydration-Mild: About 2% of water depletion	• Thirst • Decreased urine volume • Abnormally dark urine • Unexplained tiredness • Irritability • Lack of tears when crying • Headache • Dry mouth • Dizziness when standing due to orthostatic hypotension • May cause insomnia.
Moderate: About 5% -6%of water depletion	• Grogginess or sleepiness • Headache • Nausea • May feel tingling in limbs (parenthesis)
Severe: About 10% -15% of water depletion	• Muscles may become spastic • Skin may shrivel and wrinkle (decreased skin turgor) • Vision may dim • Urination will be greatly reduced and may become painful • Delirium may begin.
Over 15% of water depletion	• Usually, fatal.

COMPONENTS OF A CONDITIONING PROGRAM

WARM UP and COOL DOWN

Warming up and cooling down are very important parts of the exercise routine. There are physical and psychological benefits to both these components that can be as simple as a slow walk before and after your exercise program.

Benefits of warming up	Benefits of cooling down
<ul><li>Increases the temperature in the muscles, which increases the speed of contraction and relaxation.</li><li>Reduces premature lactic acid build up and fatigue during high level exercises.</li><li>Increases speed of nerve impulse conduction.</li><li>Increases elasticity of connective tissues</li><li>Increases muscle metabolism and oxygen consumption that enhances aerobic performance.</li><li>Alert for potential muscle injury that may arise during higher intensities.</li><li>Increases endorphins.</li><li>Allows the heart rate to get to a workable rate for beginning exercise.</li><li>Increases production of synovial fluid located between the joints to reduce friction.</li><li>Psychological warm up to mentally focus on training and competition.</li></ul>	<ul><li>Prevents venous blood pooling at the extremities, which reduces chance of dizziness or fainting.</li><li>Reduces the potential for Delayed Onset Muscle Soreness (DOMS).</li><li>Aids in removing waste products in muscles, such as lactic acid.</li><li>Reduces the level of adrenaline and other exercise hormones in the blood to lower the chance of post-exercise disturbances in cardiac rhythm.</li><li>Allows the heart to return back safely to resting rate.</li></ul>

Start out every routine with a warmup first. Here are some suggestions

- Walking or outside
- Running up and down some stairs
- Jumping jacks
- Running in place
- Dynamic stretching

Equipment

- Treadmill
- Stationary or Recumbent bike
- Stair climber or Elliptical
- Mini trampoline

Duration, Frequency, Intensity and Movement Patterns

Intensity: How *much* mental and physical *effort* it takes to sustain an activity.	This can be done using the target heart rate range THR (optimum exercise intensity levels through beats per minute, talk test or rate of perceived exertion.
Duration: How *long* the training lasts.	The higher the intensity, the shorter the duration. The American College of Sports Medicine guidelines recommends all healthy adults aged 18–65 yr should participate in moderate intensity aerobic physical activity for a minimum of 30 min on five days per week, or vigorous intensity aerobic activity for a minimum of 20 min on three days per week.
Frequency: How *often* the training occurs.	Training should be performed at least every other day or three days a week. Cardiac/aerobic conditioning can be done daily, although you may want to vary exercises. Regarding strength training, it is important to give each muscle group 48 hours to recover. Alternate upper and lower body with isolated abdomen/core exercises every other day. For those working out several days a week, find a schedule that works for you as long as you give each muscle group 48 hours of recovery time.

Movement Patterns and Examples
 	
Basic movements that help to increase overall body strengthening
	• Bend and Lift: Squats, Dead Lifts and Leg presses
	    ○ Picking up item off floor
	• Single Leg: Step ups, Single leg stance, Lunges
	    ○ Walking up steps
	• Push: Shoulder press, Bench press, Push up
	    ○ Pushing Shopping cart or Lawn mower
	• Pull: Lat pull downs, Seated rows
	    ○ Vacuuming, Raking
	• Rotational
	    ○ Shoveling snow

Diaphragmatic Breathing

• Lie either on your back with your knees bent or sit up
• Inhale through your nose; as you do so, allow your stomach to rise. Limit movement in your chest. Attempt to push your bottom ribs out to the side as you breathe in.
• Exhale through your mouth; as you do so, allow your stomach to fall. Limit movement in your chest.
• Repeat for at least 10 cycles.

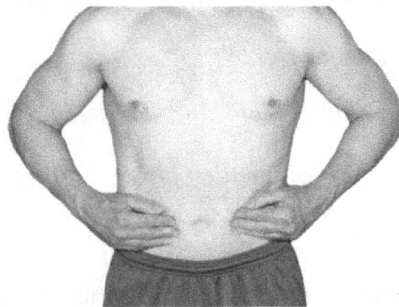

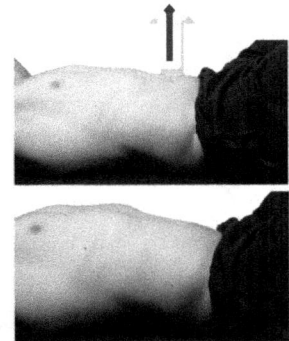

Pursed Lip Breathing

(PLB) is a breathing technique that consists of inhaling through the nose with the mouth closed and then exhaling through tightly pressed (pursed) lips. This technique is frequently in those with cardiac or respiratory issues.   *"Smell the Roses then Blow Out the Candle".*

Breathing with Exercise

Exhale on the exertion. For example, exhale when you are lying on your back and pushing a weight up or when bending your arm doing a bicep curl,. Inhale as you bring the weight slowly to your chest or when you straighten your arm with a bicep curl..

ANATOMY

ANATOMICAL POSITIONS and PLANES

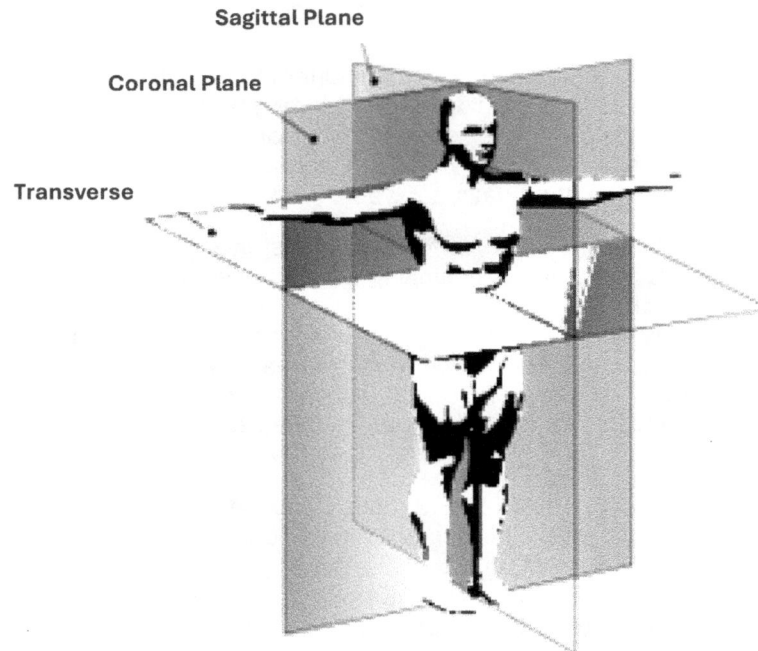

Anterior – Towards the front of the body.

Posterior – Towards the back of the body.

Distal – Away from the body or any point of reference, or from the point of attachment or origin.

Proximal – Closer to the body or any point of reference, or to the point of attachment or origin.

Medial – Situated towards the midline of the body.

Lateral – Position farther from the midline of the body.

Inferior – Away from the head or lower surface of a structure.

Superior – Towards the head or situated above.

Transverse /Axial / Horizontal plane is parallel to the ground, which separates the superior from the inferior or the head from the feet.

Coronal / Frontal/Frontal plane is perpendicular to the ground, which separates the anterior from the posterior or the front from the back

Sagittal / Lateral plane is a Y-Z plane, perpendicular to the ground, which separates left from right.

Upper Extremity (UE): Shoulders, Chest, Arms, Hands, etc

Lower Extremity (LE): Hips, Legs, Ankle Foot , etc

ANATOMICAL DIRECTIONS

Range of Motion (ROM): The distance and direction a joint can move between the flexed and extended position (*see flexion and extension below*). This can also be the act of attempting to increase the distance through therapeutic exercise and/or stretching for physiological gain.

Flexion - Bending movement that decreases the angle between two parts. Bending the knee or elbow are examples of flexion. Flexion of the hip or shoulder moves the limb forward (towards the front of the body).

Extension - The opposite of flexion; a straightening movement that increases the angle between body parts. The knees are extended when standing up. When straightening the arm, the elbow is extended. Extension of the hip or shoulder moves the limb backward (towards the back of the body).

Hyperextension – Extending the joint beyond extension.

Abduction - A lateral movement that pulls a structure or part away from the midline of the body. Raising the arms to the sides is an example of abduction.

Adduction - A medial movement that pulls a structure or part towards the midline of the body, or towards the midline of a limb. Dropping the arms to the sides, or bringing the knees together, are examples of adduction.

Internal rotation (or *medial rotation*). Inward rotary movement around the axis of the bone. Internal rotation of the shoulder or hip would point the toes or the flexed forearm inwards (towards the midline).

External rotation (or *lateral rotation*). External rotary movement around the axis of the bone. It would turn the toes or the flexed forearm outwards (away from the midline).

Elevation - Movement in a superior direction. Shrugging or bringing the shoulders up is an example of elevation.

Depression - Movement in an inferior direction, the opposite of elevation. Pushing the shoulders down is an example of depression.

Pronation - Internal rotation the hand or foot to face downward or posterior. Pronating the foot is a combination of eversion and abduction.

Supination - External rotation of the hand or foot to face upward or anterior. Raising the inside or medial margin of the foot.

Dorsiflexion – Movement at the ankle of the foot superiorly towards the shin. The up position of tapping the foot.

Plantarflexion – Movement at the ankle of the foot inferiorly away from the shin. Pointing the foot downward.

Eversion – Moving the sole of the foot away from the median plane or outward.

Inversion - Moving the sole of the foot towards the median plane or inward.

Ipsilateral – Same side of the body

Contralateral – Opposite side of the body

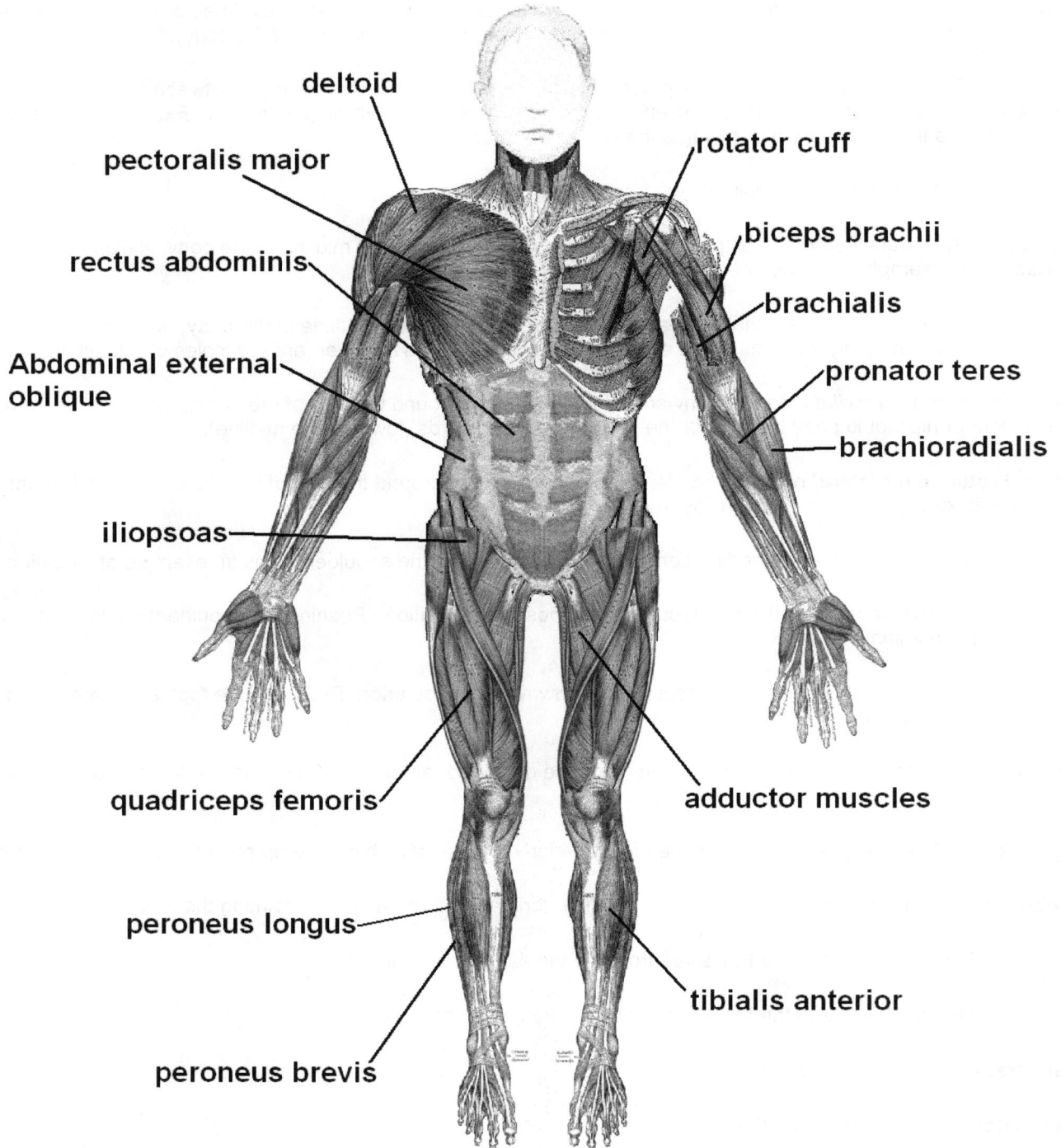

MUSCLES

Grey's Anatomy

ANTERIOR

deltoid

pectoralis major

rectus abdominis

Abdominal external oblique

iliopsoas

quadriceps femoris

peroneus longus

peroneus brevis

rotator cuff

biceps brachii

brachialis

pronator teres

brachioradialis

adductor muscles

tibialis anterior

Muscle Name (AKA)	Joint Action
Pectoralis major	Shoulder flexion, adduction, internal rotation
Deltoid (anterior)	Shoulder abduction, flexion, internal rotation
Rotator cuff (SITS) Supraspinatus Infraspinatus Teres minor Subscapularis	Shoulder: Supraspinatus: Abduction Infraspinatus: External rotation Teres minor: External rotation Subscapularis: Internal rotation
Biceps brachii	Elbow flexion; Forearm supination
Brachialis	Elbow flexion
Pronator teres	Elbow flexion; Forearm pronation
Brachioradialis	Elbow flexion
Tensor fasciae latae	Hip flexion, medial rotation & abduction
Gracilis*	Hip adduction & internal rotation;Knee flexion & internal rotation
Adductor muscles Adductor magnus, longus & brevis	Hip adduction
Tibialis anterior	Ankle dorsiflexion; foot inversion
Peroneus brevis	Ankle plantarflexion; Foot eversion
Peroneus longus	Ankle plantarflexion; Foot eversion
Rectus femoris (quadriceps femoris)	Hip extension (esp. when knee is extended); Knee flexion
Vastus medialis	Knee extension (esp. when hip is flexed)
Vastus lateralis	Knee extension (esp. when hip is flexed)
Sartorius	Hip flexion & external rotation; Knee flexion & internal rotation
Pectineus	Hip adduction
Iliopsoas, Psosas, Iliacus	Hip flexion & external rotation
Abdominal external oblique	Trunk lateral flexion
Rectus abdominis	Trunk flexion & lateral flexion
Abdominal internal oblique	Trunk lateral flexion

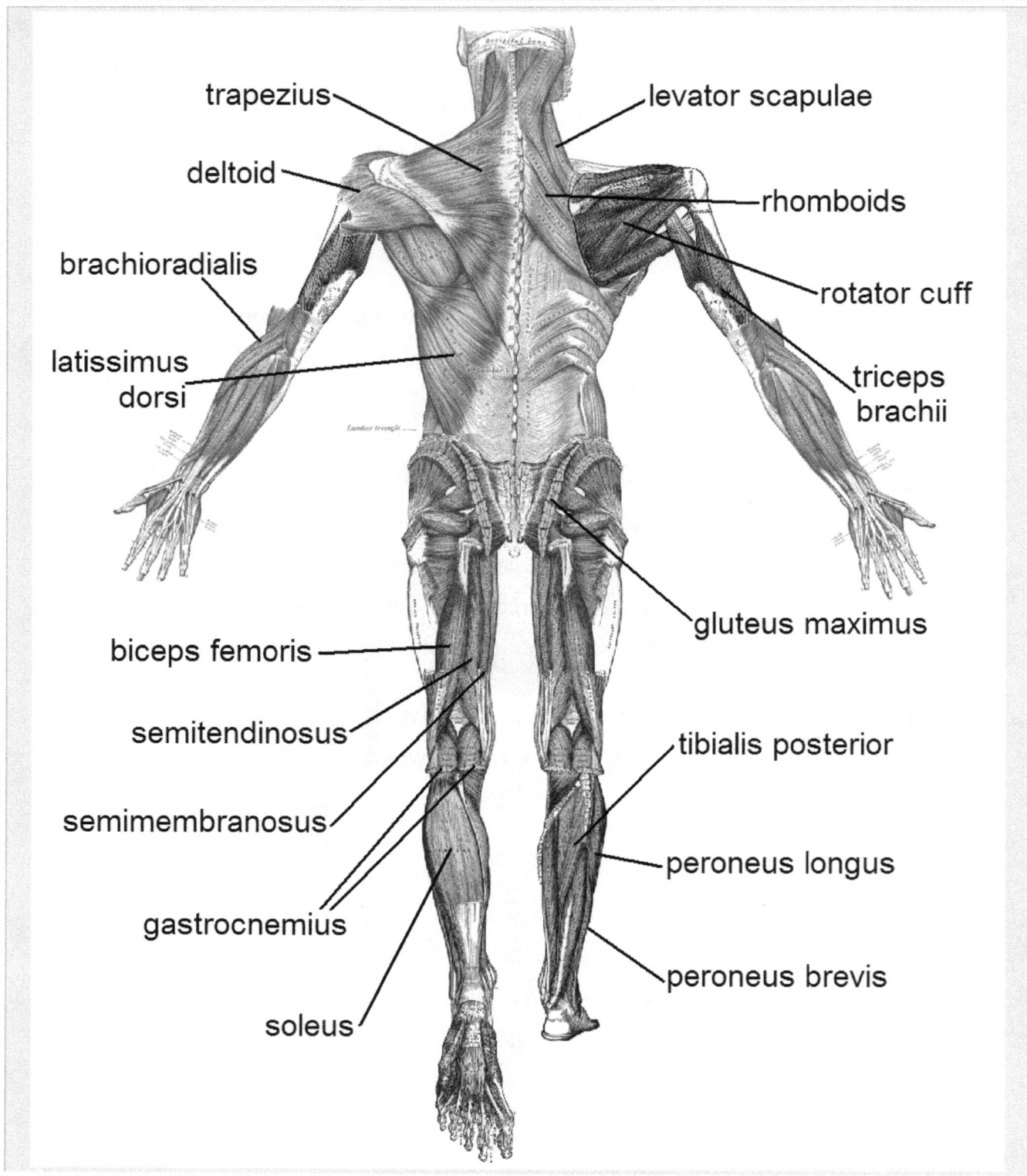

MUSCLES

Grey's Anatomy

POSTERIOR

trapezius

levator scapulae

deltoid

rhomboids

brachioradialis

rotator cuff

latissimus dorsi

triceps brachii

gluteus maximus

biceps femoris

semitendinosus

tibialis posterior

semimembranosus

peroneus longus

gastrocnemius

peroneus brevis

soleus

Muscle Name (AKA)	Joint Action
Deltoid (posterior)	Shoulder abduction, extension, external rotation
Trapezius	Scapula or Shoulder girdle:, Upper traps: Scapula elevation. Middle traps: Scapula adduction. Lower traps: Scapula depression
Levator scapulae	Scapula elevation
Rhomboids	Scapula adduction & elevation
Triceps brachii	Elbow extension
Gluteus medius	Hip abduction
Gluteus maximus	Hip extension & external rotation
Tibialis, posterior	Inversion, stabilization, assists with plantarflexion
Soleus	Ankle plantarflexion
Gastrocnemius	Knee flexion; Ankle plantarflexion
Semimembranosus	Hip extension & internal rotation; Knee flexion & internal rotation
Semitendinosus	Hip extension & internal rotation; Knee flexion & internal rotation
Biceps femoris (long head)	Hip extension & internal rotation; Knee flexion & external rotation
Latissimus dorsi	Shoulder extension, adduction, internal rotation
Erector spinae, Longissimus, Spinalis, Iliocostalis	Trunk extension, hyperextension & lateral flexion Deep muscle that originate in the posterior iliac crest & sacrum running up the spine and inserts in the transverse process of ribs
Pes anserine, Gracilis, Sartorius, Semimembranosus, Semitendinosus	Internal rotation of tibia when knee is flexed

SKELETON

ANTERIOR (FRONT)

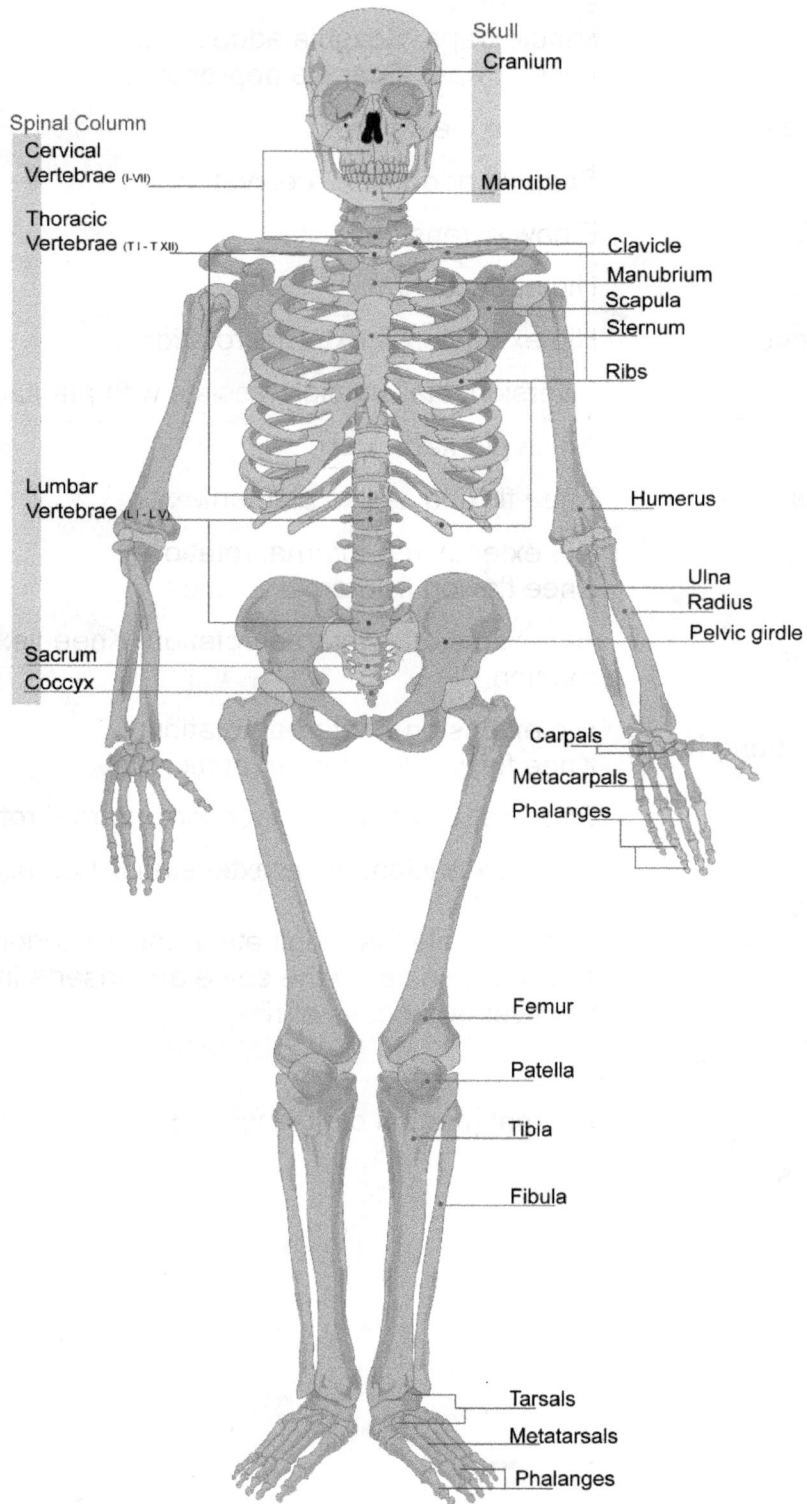

Skull
Cranium

Spinal Column
Cervical
Vertebrae (I-VII)

Thoracic
Vertebrae (T I - T XII)

Mandible

Clavicle
Manubrium
Scapula
Sternum

Ribs

Lumbar
Vertebrae (L I - L V)

Humerus

Ulna
Radius
Pelvic girdle

Sacrum
Coccyx

Carpals
Metacarpals
Phalanges

Femur

Patella

Tibia

Fibula

Tarsals
Metatarsals
Phalanges

SKELETON

POSTERIOR (BACK)

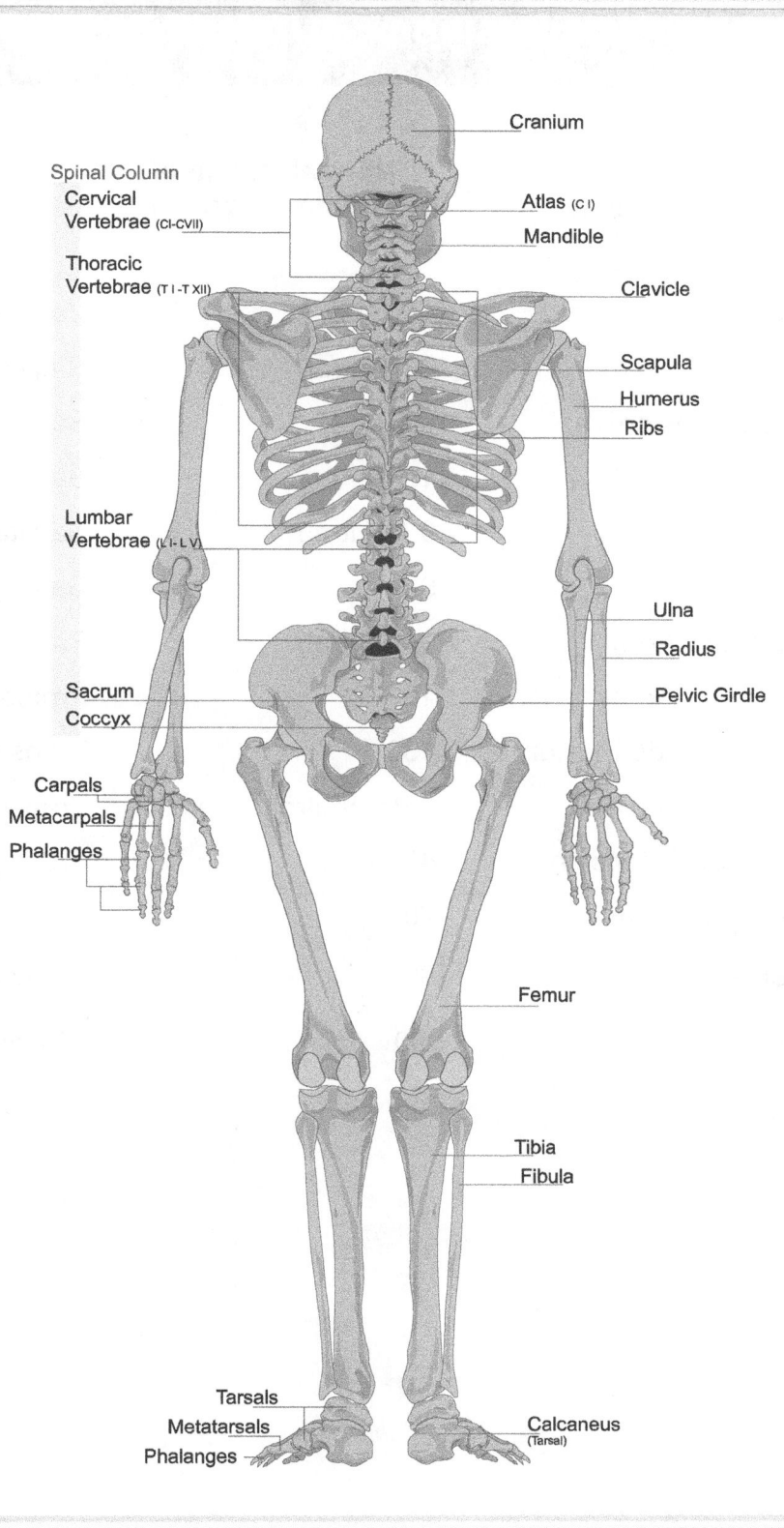

Cranium

Spinal Column
Cervical
Vertebrae (CI-CVII)

Atlas (C I)

Mandible

Thoracic
Vertebrae (T I -T XII)

Clavicle

Scapula

Humerus

Ribs

Lumbar
Vertebrae (LI-L V)

Ulna

Radius

Sacrum

Coccyx

Pelvic Girdle

Carpals

Metacarpals

Phalanges

Femur

Tibia

Fibula

Tarsals

Metatarsals

Phalanges

Calcaneus
(Tarsal)

Average Joint Range of Motion

Anatomical Positions – Upper Extremity

Joint UPPER EXTREMITY	Movement	Normal Range of Motion (degrees)	Plane
Elbow	Flexion	150	Sagittal
	Extension	0 (neutral)	Sagittal
	Hyperextension	< 10	Sagittal
Shoulder	Flexion	180	Sagittal
	Extension	0 (neutral)	Sagittal
	Hyperextension	60	Sagittal
	Adduction (Add)	0 (neutral)	Frontal
	Abduction (Abd)	180	Frontal
	Horizontal Add/Flexion	130	Transverse
	Horizontal Abd	0 (to neutral)	Transverse
	Horizontal Extension	45	Transverse
	Internal rotation	70	Sagittal
	External rotation	90	Sagittal
Radioulnar	Pronation	90	Transverse
	Supination	90	Transverse

Average Joint Range of Motion

Anatomical Positions – Lower Extremity

Joint LOWER EXTREMITY	Movement	Normal Range of Motion (degrees)	Plane
Knee	Flexion	135	Sagittal
	Extension	0 (neutral)	Sagittal
	Hyperextension	10	Sagittal
Hip	Flexion	120	Sagittal
	Extension	0 (neutral)	Sagittal
	Hyperextension	< 20	Sagittal
	Adduction (Add)	0 (neutral)	Frontal
	Abduction (Abd)	50	Frontal
	Internal rotation	40	Transverse
	External rotation	50	Transverse
Ankle	Dorsiflexion	20	Sagittal
	Plantarflexion	50	Sagittal

EQUIPMENT used in this Book.

Don't buy a lot of equipment before knowing what your goals are.

Stability / Exercise Ball Bosu

These can replace an exercise bench if you do not have the space. It is also used for many of the core strengthening exercises

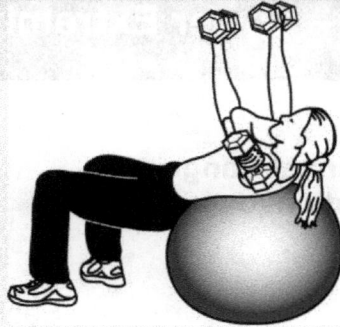

Should be inflated so that when you sit on it you are at a 90-degree angle.

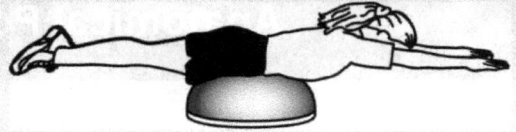

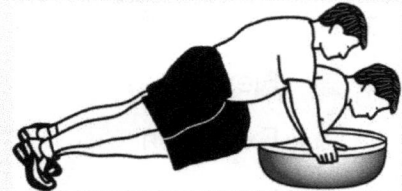

Dumbbells

Kettle Bell (optional)

Dowel with/without weight

These will be needed for your strength exercises. See *Strengthening* section on for resistance.

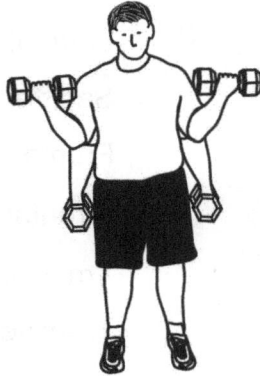

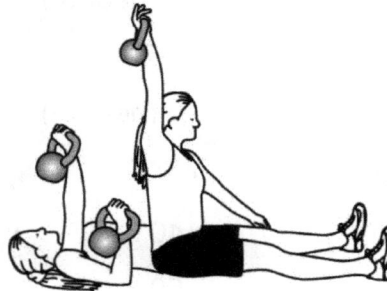

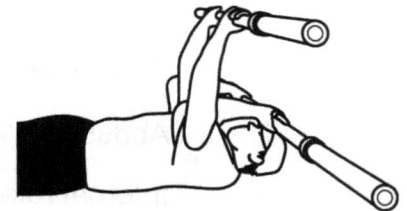

Resistance bands

In different weights/ resistance.

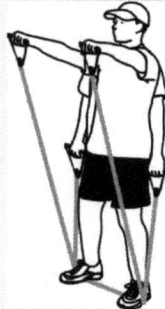

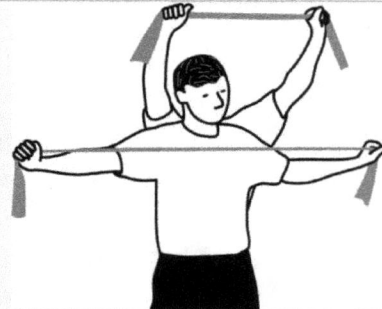

Agility Equipment

Cone hurdles, Speed hurdles, Agility ladder/rings/poles, Bosu, Stair step, Jump rope.

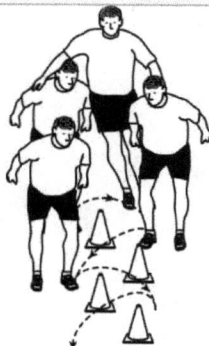

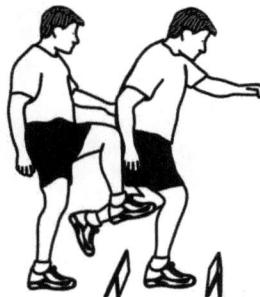

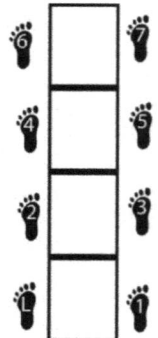

Balance Equipment

Can include
Foam rollers
(also see Myofascial below)

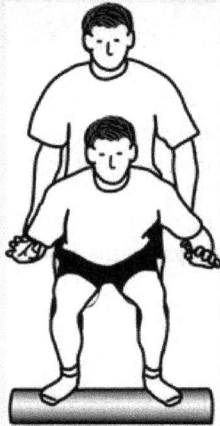

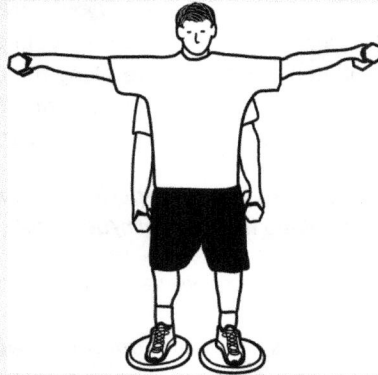

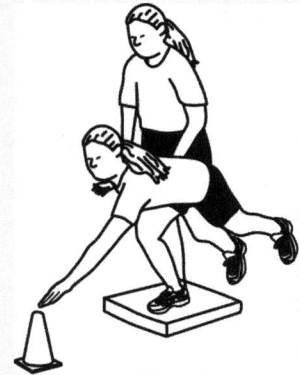

Balance discs
Balance pad
Cones
Stepper
Bosu

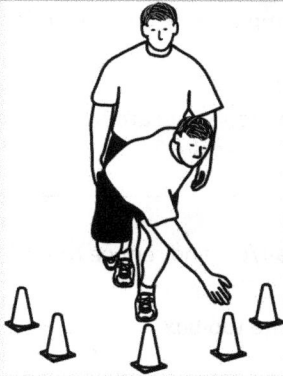

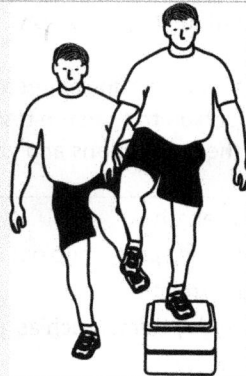

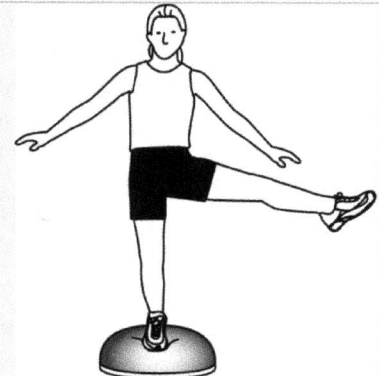

Exercise Bench (Optional)

The type really depends on what you will use it for. You can get a plain bench just for support (as above you can use a stability ball) or you can get all the bells and whistles. Some have pieces for leg extensions and curls, as well as arm pieces for butterflies. If you do not already have one, I suggest waiting until you start your exercise program and see what you feel you will need to advance.

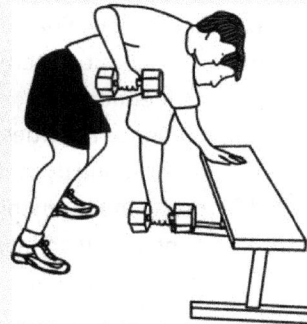

Examples For Myofascial

Massage Ball

Foam/Textured Rollers *(also see balance)*

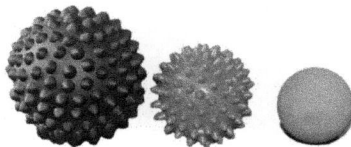

Full Rollers

Half Roller with Flat Bottom

Not Shown

- Exercise mat for floor exercises
- Ankle Weights
- Bed, couch or high table/mat
- Chair with/without arms - High or Low

- 10-inch play ball
- Pillow
- Towel roll
- Strap for stretches

SELF TESTS

Before starting the exercise program, it is a good idea to see where your baseline is. Taking the following tests will help guide you in the level you will need to start, and help progress by retaking the test periodically. *It is suggested to get a partner to help with both timing and safety, especially with balance tests.* The first 6 tests are modified versions starting at age 60 but are great for adults of any age. Tests 7-10 will help determine how quickly you can advance your balance program.

As with the exercises in this book, these tests should also be performed by those that are otherwise healthy with no chronic or acute ailments OR with supervision of a qualified health coach/personal trainer/physical therapist.

Tests 1-6 should be conducted in the following order if you are doing them at the same time.

A general warm up should be done prior to tests (*see Warm up/Cool down*).
- Stop immediately if any adverse reactions, such as nausea, dizziness, blurred vision, pain of any kind, chest pain, confusion or loss of muscle control.
- Stay hydrated, and do not proceed with testing on days with high temperature/humidity or any other conditions where you would not normally exercise.
- Practice each test several times before attempting to get an accurate score.
- It is advised that you have a second person to time the tests and make sure you are following proper form. Make sure your partner also understands the precautions and goals of these tests.

1. 30 second chair stand - Lower body strength
   - Needed for stair climbing, walking getting up out of tub/chair/car and reduce the risk of falls
2. 30 second arm curl test – Upper body strength
   - Needed to lift and carry everyday items, such as groceries and toolbox
3. 2-minute step test – Aerobic endurance
   - Needed for activities that require endurance, such as walking distance, grocery shopping and climbing stairs
4. Chair sit and reach – Lower body flexibility
   - Needed for normal gait patterns, correct posture, getting in/out of car/tub
5. Back stretch test – Shoulder flexibility
   - Needed to do various activities, such as combing hair and putting on overhead garments
6. 8 foot get up and go – Agility and dynamic balance
   - Needed for pretty much anything you do that requires getting up and walking, such as go to kitchen, bathroom or answering phone.
7. Narrow stance – Balance progression
8. Staggered stance – Balance progression
9. Tandem stance – Balance progression
10. One leg standing – Balance progression

TEST AND PURPOSE	PICTURE	EQUIPMENT NEEDED	EXPLANATION	RESULTS
30 Second Chair Stand Assess lower body strength *May not want to perform if any chronic pain or back issues. *If you are tall and have had a recent hip replacement skip this or use taller chair.		Straight back or folding chair (~17 inch height) against wall. Stopwatch, wrist watch or clock within view with second hand	*Sit with feet flat on the floor and arms crossed over the chest. *Get up to a full stand and then sit back down. ** Start the time – Immediately repeat as many *full stands* as you can in 30 seconds. *If you cannot stand with hands over chest, try pushing off on your thighs or get a chair with arms and push off arms. If using assist, make sure you note this for progression.*	**Normal Range repetitions** <table><tr><td>Age</td><td>Men</td><td>Women</td></tr><tr><td>60-64</td><td>14-19</td><td>12-17</td></tr><tr><td>65-69</td><td>12-18</td><td>11-16</td></tr><tr><td>70-74</td><td>12-17</td><td>10-15</td></tr><tr><td>75-79</td><td>11-17</td><td>10-15</td></tr><tr><td>80-84</td><td>10-15</td><td>9-14</td></tr><tr><td>85-89</td><td>8-14</td><td>8-13</td></tr><tr><td>90-94</td><td>7-12</td><td>4-11</td></tr></table>

Normal Range repetitions (30 Second Chair Stand)

Age	Men	Women
60-64	14-19	12-17
65-69	12-18	11-16
70-74	12-17	10-15
75-79	11-17	10-15
80-84	10-15	9-14
85-89	8-14	8-13
90-94	7-12	4-11

TEST AND PURPOSE	PICTURE	EQUIPMENT NEEDED	EXPLANATION	RESULTS
30 Second Arm Curl Test Upper body strength		Straight back or folding chair without arms. Can be done in standing. Stopwatch or clock within view with second hand Women: 5 lb dumbbell Men: 8 lb dumbbell Can use a wrist weight if arthritis and cannot hold a dumbbell	*Sit with feet flat on the floor towards the edge seat towards dominant side. **Start with the arm extended by your side holding dumbbell in the dominant hand. *Bend elbow with palm facing you keeping the upper arm next to the body (elbow pressed into your side). *Return to starting position. *Keep the wrist straight – do not flex or extend the wrist. **Start the time – Immediately repeat as many arm curls as you can in 30 seconds *with proper form.* *If you cannot hold the suggested weight with proper form, use a lighter weight. Make sure you note this for progression.*	**Normal Range repetitions**

Normal Range repetitions (30 Second Arm Curl Test)

Age	Men	Women
60-64	16-22	13-19
65-69	15-21	12-18
70-74	14-21	12-17
75-79	13-19	11-17
80-84	13-19	10-16
85-89	11-17	10-15
90-94	10-14	8-13

TEST AND PURPOSE	PICTURE	EQUIPMENT NEEDED	EXPLANATION	RESULTS
2 Minute Step Test Aerobic endurance		Wall for support and to mark step height. Sturdy chair to hold on opposite side if unsteady. Stopwatch or clock within view with second hand	*For accuracy, may need a second person to judge step height and count. *Step with side next to wall. Bring knee up mid-thigh between the knee and the hip. Mark the wall with tape at this height. This will be your minimum step height. *Practice marching in place to this step height. **Start the time – Immediately start marching (not jogging) for 2 minutes. Count the number of *full steps* (both legs) that come up to step height. Every time the right knee reaches proper step height; this is counted as one step. *If shortness of breath, extreme fatigue or unable to continue to step height, stop test and this is your baseline. * If unable to get to step height, but able to complete 2 minutes. Make sure you note this for progression. *If unsteady, hold onto chair on opposite side for support.*	**Normal Range steps** See table below

Normal Range steps

Age	Men	Women
60-64	87-115	75-107
65-69	86-116	73-107
70-74	80-110	68-101
75-79	73-109	68-100
80-84	71-103	60-90
85-89	59-91	55-85
90-94	52-86	44-72

TEST AND PURPOSE	PICTURE	EQUIPMENT NEEDED	EXPLANATION	RESULTS
Chair Sit And Reach Lower body flexibility, *primarily hamstrings* *Do not do if recent hip replacement or severe osteoporosis. *Stretch to discomfort, not pain.		Chair (~17 inch height). Make sure chair is secure and does not tip forward. 18 inch ruler or yardstick	*Sit on the edge chair – you should feel the middle of the thigh at the edge of the chair. *Bend one leg with foot flat on floor. *Straighten the target leg in front with heel on the floor and foot flexed up. *Reach forward with one hand over the other and middle fingers even. *Exhale as you bend forward at the hips and reach forward towards or past the toes. Keep the extended knee straight and adjust if it bends. *Practice a few times on both legs to see which one you would prefer for testing. Do two tests and measure as below. **Measure tips of middle fingers to the tip of the shoe (closest to ½ inch). ***The midpoint at the toe of the shoe is considered zero (0), and is scored as such if you reach this point. ***If the reach is short, score this as a minus (-) ***If the reach is past this point, score this as a plus (+)	**Normal Range inches** | Age	Men	Women | |---|---|---| | 60-64 | -2.5 +4.0 | -0.5 + 5.0 | | 65-69 | -3.0 +3.0 | -0.5 + 4.5 | | 70-74 | -3.0 +3.0 | -1.0 + 4.0 | | 75-79 | -4.0 +2.0 | -1.5 + 3.5 | | 80-84 | -5.5 +1.5 | 2.0 + 3.0 | | 85-89 | -5.5 +0.5 | -2.5 + 2.5 | | 90-94 | -6.5 -0.5 | -4.5 + 1.0 |

Normal Range inches (Chair Sit And Reach):

Age	Men	Women
60-64	-2.5 / +4.0	-0.5 / + 5.0
65-69	-3.0 / +3.0	-0.5 / + 4.5
70-74	-3.0 / +3.0	-1.0 / + 4.0
75-79	-4.0 / +2.0	-1.5 / + 3.5
80-84	-5.5 / +1.5	2.0 / + 3.0
85-89	-5.5 / +0.5	-2.5 / + 2.5
90-94	-6.5 / -0.5	-4.5 / + 1.0

TEST AND PURPOSE	PICTURE	EQUIPMENT NEEDED	EXPLANATION	RESULTS
Back Stretch Test Shoulder flexibility *Do not do if any upper back, shoulder or neck injuries		18-inch ruler or yardstick	*Will need second person to measure. *Stand and place the target arm over the same shoulder, palm down with fingers extended. Reach down the middle of the back. *Place the opposite arm around the back, palm up reaching up the middle of the back towards other hand. Try to touch middle fingers together or overlap if possible. *Do not overlap fingers and pull.* *Practice a few times on both arms to see which one you would prefer for testing. Do two tests and measure as below. **Measure the distance between tips of middle fingers or overlap. ***If the middle fingers do not touch, score this as a minus (-) ***If the middle fingers just touch, score this as a zero (0) ***If the middle fingers overlap, score this as a plus (+)	**Normal Range inches**

Normal Range inches (Back Stretch Test):

Age	Men	Women
60-64	-6.5 / +0.0	-3.0 / + 1.5
65-69	-7.5 / -1.0	-3.5 / + 1.5
70-74	-8.0 / -1.0	-4.0 / + 1.0
75-79	-9.0 / -2.0	-5.0 / + 0.5
80-84	-9.5 / -2.0	-5.5 / + 0.0
85-89	-9.5 / -3.0	-7.0 / -1.0
90-94	-10.5 / -4.0	-8.0 / -1.0

TEST AND PURPOSE	PICTURE	EQUIPMENT NEEDED	EXPLANATION	RESULTS		
8 Foot Get Up And Go Agility and dynamic balance *If unsteady, have someone by your side in case you lose your balance.	 8 feet →	Chair against wall (~17-inch height) Cone or another marker to walk around Stopwatch or clock within view with second hand *Put chair against wall and cone 8 feet in front. Measure from front of chair to back of cone (side facing chair).	*This is done better with a partner watching the clock or a stopwatch. *Sit on chair, back straight, feet flat on floor, one foot slightly in front, torso leaning slightly forward and hands resting on thighs. **Start the time – Immediately get up and walk around the cone (either side) and return to chair. Stopwatch immediately when seated. **Try 2-3x and record the fastest time within 10th /second. *Can use a cane or walker or start from standing position. Make sure you note this for progression.	Normal Range seconds		

				Normal Range seconds		
				Age	Men	Women
				60-64	5.6-3.8	6.0-4.4
				65-69	5.9-4.3	6.4-4.8
				70-74	6.2-4.4	7.1-4.9
				75-79	7.2-4.6	7.4-5.2
				80-84	7.6-5.2	8.7-5.7
				85-89	8.9-5.5	9.6-6.2
				90-94	10.0-6.2	11.5-7.3

TEST AND PURPOSE	PICTURE	EQUIPMENT NEEDED	EXPLANATION	RESULTS
Narrow Stance Balance progression		Wall, counter or chair within arm's reach for support if needed Stopwatch or clock within view with second hand	Keep your feet together and stand for up to one minute. *Time stops if loss of balance with need to hold on to support.	One minute: Normal *Progress to Staggered Stance Test* *Less than 30 seconds: Continue balance program with wider stance and progress to narrow stance using support. *(See Balance)*
Staggered Stance Balance progression		Wall, counter or chair within arm's reach for support if needed Stopwatch or clock within view with second hand	Stand with one foot in front of the other and slightly off to the side. Stand for up to one minute. Repeat on other side for comparison *Time stops if loss of balance with need to hold on to support.	One minute: Normal *Progress to Tandem Stance Test* *Less than 30 seconds: Continue balance program using support. *(See Balance)*
Tandem Stance Balance progression		Wall, counter or chair within arm's reach for support if needed Stopwatch or clock within view with second hand	Stand with one foot directly in back of the other – toe should be touching the opposite heel. Hold for up to one minute. Repeat on other side for comparison *Time stops if loss of balance with need to hold on to support.	One minute: Normal *Progress to One Leg Standing Balance* *Less than 30 seconds: Continue balance program using support. *(See Balance)*
Single Leg Stance Balance progression		Wall, counter or chair within arm's reach for support if needed Stopwatch or clock within view with second hand	Stand on one leg for up to one minute. Repeat on other side for comparison *Time stops if loss of balance with need to hold on to support or if opposite foot taps the floor	One minute: Normal *Less than 30 seconds: Continue balance program using support. *(See Balance)*

EXERCISE Myofascial Release	EXERCISE NUMBER	PAGE	REPS	SETS	X DAY	HOLD
ANTERIOR CHEST - BALL	1					
ANTERIOR CHEST - FOAM ROLL	2					
LATISSIMUS DORSI – BALL	3					
LATISSIMUS DORSI - FOAM ROLL	4					
TRICEP – FOAM ROLL	5					
OCCIPITAL RELEASE - FOAM ROLL	6					
THORACIC MOBILIZATION – SUPINE - FOAM ROLL	7					
THORACIC MOBILIZATION – STANDING - FOAM ROLL	8					
LUMBAR – STANDING – BALL - can do with foam roll	9					
LUMBAR – SUPINE – FOAM ROLLER	10					
HIP FLEXORS - BALL	11					
HIP FLEXORS – FOAM ROLL	12					
QUADRICEPS – BILATERAL - FOAM ROLL	13					
QUADRICEP – SINGLE - FOAM ROLL	14					
GLUTE /PIRIFORMIS - FOAM ROLL	15					
HIP ADDUCTORS – FOAM ROLL	16					
HAMSTRING – BILATERAL - FOAM ROLL	17					
HAMSTRING – SINGLE – FOAM ROLL	18					
CALVES – BILATERAL - FOAM ROLL	19					
CALVES – SINGLE - FOAM ROLL	20					
ILIOTIBIAL BAND (IT Band) - FOAM ROLL	21					
ILIOTIBIAL BAND (IT Band) - BALL	22					
PLANTAR FASCIA ROLLING – BALL	23					
PLANTAR FASCIA ROLLING - COLD SODA CAN	24					

EXERCISE **Flexibility (Stretching)**	EXERCISE NUMBER	PAGE	REPS	SETS	X DAY	HOLD
INVERSION	1					
EVERSION	2					
ANTERIOR TIBIALIS	3					
PLANTARFLEXION	4					
DORSIFLEXION - STRAP	5					
DORSIFLEXION - FLOOR ASSISTED	6					
STANDING CALF STRETCH - GASTROC	7					
STANDING CALF STRETCH - GASTROC – HAND ON KNEE	8					
GASTROCNEMIUS STAIR STRETCH	9					
STANDING CALF STRETCH - SOLEUS	10					
HAMSTRING STRETCH – TOWEL, BAND, STRAP or BELT	11					
HAMSTRING STRETCH – TOWEL, BAND, STRAP or BELT	12					
HAMSTRING STRETCH - TABLE, BED OR COUCH	13					
HAMSTRING / KNEE EXTENSION STRETCH - SEATED	14					
HAMSTRING STRETCH - STANDING	15					
TOE TOUCH – STANDING - NARROW or WIDE BOS	16					
HEEL SLIDES - SELF ASSISTED	17					
HEEL SLIDES - LONG SIT ASSISTED - TOWEL, BAND, STRAP or BELT	18					
HEEL SLIDES - SUPINE	19					
KNEE BENDS - EXERCISE BALL	20					
KNEE FLEXION – SELF ASSISTED - PRONE	21					
KNEE FLEXION – BELT ASSISTED - PRONE	22					
HEEL SLIDES - SELF ASSISTED	23					
HEEL SLIDES - SEATED	24					
KNEE FLEXION – SCOOT FORWARD - SEATED	25					

EXERCISE **Flexibility (Stretching)**	EXERCISE NUMBER	PAGE	REPS	SETS	X DAY	HOLD
KNEE FLEXION – STAIR OR STEP	26					
PIRIFORMIS STRETCH	27					
PIRIFORMIS STRETCH - EXERCISE BALL	28					
PIRIFORMIS STRETCH - LONG SIT	29					
PIRIFORMIS STRETCH – STANDING	30					
HIP FLEXOR STRETCH - SIDE OF BALL or CHAIR	31					
HIP FLEXOR STRETCH - STANDING	32					
HIP FLEXOR STRETCH - HALF KNEEL	33					
RUNNER'S STRETCH - MODIFIED	34					
HIP FLEXOR STRETCH – SUPINE	35					
HIP FLEXOR STRETCH – SUPINE - 2	36					
QUAD STRETCH - SIDELYING	37					
QUAD STRETCH - STANDING	38					
KNEE FALL OUT STRETCH or FROG STRETCH	39					
BUTTERFLY STRETCH	40					
HIP ADDUCTOR STRECH – KNEELING	41					
HIP ADDUCTOR STRECH - STANDING	42					
HIP EXTERNAL ROTATION STRETCH - SUPINE	43					
HIP INTERNAL ROTATION STRETCH - SEATED	44					
IT BAND STRETCH - STANDING	45					
IT BAND STRETCH -- SIDELYING	46					
NECK ROTATION and SIDE BENDS	47					
NECK FLEXION AND EXTENSION	48					
TRUNK FLEXION - SEATED	49					
LOW BACK STRETCH - SEATED	50					
LOW BACK STRETCH – STANDING - STRAIGHT & LATERAL	51					
LOW BACK STRETCH – RAIL OR DOORKNOB	52					

EXERCISE **Flexibility (Stretching)**	EXERCISE NUMBER	PAGE	REPS	SETS	X DAY	HOLD
PRAYER STRETCH and LATERAL	53					
PRAYER STRETCH - EXERCISE BALL	54					
CAT AND CAMEL	55					
KNEE TO CHEST STRETCH - SINGLE and BILATERAL	56					
PRONE ON ELBOWS	57					
PRESS UPS	58					
TRUNK ROTATION STRETCH – SINGLE LEG	59					
LOWER TRUNK ROTATIONS – BILATERAL	60					
TRUNK ROTATION - SEATED	61					
TRUNK ROTATION - STANDING or SEATED – DOWEL	62					
LATERAL TRUNK STRETCH - SINGLE, SEATED or STANDING	63					
LATERAL TRUNK STRETCH - BILATERAL SEATED or STANDING	64					
FLEXION - SUPINE - DOWEL	65					
WALL WALK	66					
FLEXION - TABLE SLIDE	67					
FLEXION - TABLE SLIDE - BALL	68					
EXTERNAL ROTATION - SUPINE – DOWEL *INTERNAL ROTATION ON OPPOSITE ARM*	69					
EXTERNAL ROTATION - 90-90 - DOWEL	70					
EXTERNAL ROTATION – SEATED – DOWEL *INTERNAL ROTATION ON OPPOSITE ARM*	71					
EXTERNAL ROTATION – STANDING – DOWEL *INTERNAL ROTATION ON OPPOSITE ARM*	72					
ABDUCTION - TABLE SLIDE - BALL	75					
ABDUCTION WITH DOWEL	76					
LYING DOWN EXTENSION - TABLE or BED	77					
WAND EXTENSION - STANDING	78					
CHEST STRETCH – SEATED, STANDING, or SUPINE	79					

EXERCISE Flexibility (Stretching)	EXERCISE NUMBER	PAGE	REPS	SETS	X DAY	HOLD
TRICEP STRETCH - STRAP or TOWEL	82					
POSTERIOR SHOULDER/DELTOID RELEASE	83					
POSTERIOR CAPSULE STRETCH	84					

Worksheets

EXERCISE Core / Stability	EXERCISE NUMBER	PAGE	REPS	SETS	X DAY	HOLD
ABDOMINAL BRACING TRAINING	1					
ABDOMINAL BRACING - SUPINE	2					
PELVIC TILT - SUPINE	3					
PELVIC TILT - KNEELING	4					
BRIDGING	5					
BRIDGE - BOSU	6					
BRIDGING WITH PILLOW SQUEEZE	7					
BRIDGING WITH PILLOW SQUEEZE - BOSU	8					
BRACE SUPINE MARCHING / BRIDGE LEG UP	9					
BRIDGE LEG UP - BOSU -	10					
SINGLE LEG BRIDGE	11					
BRIDGE SINGLE LEG - BOSU	12					
BRIDGING CROSSED LEG	13					
BRIDGING CROSSED LEG – BOSU	14					
BRIDGING CROSSED LEG - ARMS UP	15					
BRIDGING CROSSED LEG - ARMS UP - BOSU	16					
BRIDGE - ELASTIC BAND	17					
BRIDGING - ABDUCTION - ELASTIC BAND	18					
FLOOR BRIDGE - EXERCISE BALL	19					
FLOOR BRIDGE ALTERNATE LEG LIFT - EXERCISE BALL	20					
BRIDGE UPPER BACK - EXERCISE BALL	21					
BRIDGE UPPER BACK - SINGLE LEG - EXERCISE BALL	22					
QUADRUPED ALTERNATE ARM	23					
QUADRUPED ALTERNATE LEG	24					
QUADRUPED ALTERNATE ARM AND LEG	25					
BIRD DOG ELBOW TOUCHES	26					

EXERCISE Core / Stability	EXERCISE NUMBER	PAGE	REPS	SETS	X DAY	HOLD
PRONE BALL	27					
PRONE BALL - ALTERNATE ARM	28					
PRONE BALL - ALTERNATE LEG	29					
PRONE BALL - ALTERNATE ARM AND LEG	30					
MODIFIED PLANK	31					
MODIFIED PLANK - ALTERNATE LEG	32					
FULL PLANK	33					
PLANK - ALTERNATE ARMS	34					
PLANK - ALTERNATE LEGS	35					
PLANK - EXERCISE BALL	36					
PRONE ON ELBOWS	37					
PRESS UPS	38					
SKYDIVER	39					
PRONE SUPERMAN - BOSU	40					
TRUNK EXTENSION - BOSU	41					
TRUNK EXTENSION - HANDS CROSSED IN FRONT - BOSU	43					
SUPERMAN - ARMS BACK- EXERCISE BALL	44					
SUPERMAN – BOTH ARMS IN FRONT - EXERCISE BALL	45					
SUPERMAN – ONE ARM FORWARD / ONE ARM BACK - EXERCISE BALL	46					
LATERAL PLANK MODIFIED	47					
LATERAL PLANK MODIFIED- BOSU	48					
LATERAL PLANK - 1 KNEE 1 FOOT	49					
LATERAL PLANK - 1 KNEE 1 FOOT – BOSU	50					
LATERAL PLANK	51					
LATERAL PLANK - BOSU	52					

EXERCISE	EXERCISE NUMBER	PAGE	REPS	SETS	X DAY	HOLD
Core / Stability						
LEAN BACK	53					
LEAN BACK - BOSU	54					
LEAN BACK WITH ARMS OUT	55					
LEAN BACK WITH ARMS OUT - BOSU	56					
LEAN BACK WITH TWIST	57					
LEAN BACK WITH TWIST – BOSU	58					
CRUNCHY FROG	59					
SEATED BIKE - FORWARD AND BACKWARDS	60					
CRUNCH – ARMS OUT	61					
CRUNCH – ARMS OUT - BOSU	62					
CRUNCH – ARMS IN BACK OF HEAD	63					
CRUNCH – ARMS IN BACK OF HEAD - BOSU	64					
OBLIQUE CRUNCH	65					
OBLIQUE CRUNCH - BOSU	66					
90 DEGREE CRUNCH	67					
BALL CRUNCH – Can put legs on seat of chair	68					
CURL UPS – ARMS ON LEGS - EXERCISE BALL	69					
CURL UPS- ARMS CROSSED IN FRONT - EXERCISE BALL	70					
CURL UPS – ARMS BEHIND HEAD - EXERCISE BALL	71					
SUPINE CRUNCH TOUCH - EXERCISE BALL	72					
LOWER ABDOMINAL CRUNCH – WITH or WITHOUT BALL	73					
HIGH MARCH CRUNCH	74					
STANDING SIDE CRUNCH	75					
STANDING BIKE CRUNCH	76					

EXERCISE Lower Extremity - Lying & Seated Strengthening and Range of Motion	EXERCISE NUMBER	PAGE	REPS	SETS	X DAY	HOLD
INVERSION – SEATED - ELASTIC BAND	1					
INVERSION – SEATED - ELASTIC BAND - 2	2					
EVERSION – SEATED - ELASTIC BAND	3					
EVERSION – SEATED - ELASTIC BAND - 2	4					
ANKLE PUMPS - SEATED	5					
ANKLE PUMPS – SUPINE or FEET UP ON STOOL	6					
DORSIFLEXION – SEATED - ELASTIC BAND	7					
DORSIFLEXION – SEATED - ELASTIC BAND - 2	8					
PLANTARFLEXION - STRAP	9					
PLANTARFLEXION - SEATED – ELASTIC BAND	10					
HEEL SLIDES - SUPINE	11					
HEEL SLIDES - RESISTED EXTENSION – ELASTIC BAND	12					
QUAD SET –ISOMETRIC	13					
QUAD SET WITH TOWEL UNDER HEEL - ISOMETRIC	14					
SHORT ARC QUAD (SAQ) – SELF ASSISTED	15					
SHORT ARC QUAD - (SAQ)	16					
KNEE EXTENSION - SELF ASSISTED	17					
PARTIAL ARC QUAD - LOW SEAT	18					
LONG ARC QUAD (LAQ) – LOW SEAT (90 deg)	19					
LONG ARC QUAD (LAQ) – LOW SEAT - ANKLE WEIGHTS	20					
LONG ARC QUAD (LAQ) - HIGH SEAT	21					
LONG ARC QUAD (LAQ) - HIGH SEAT - ANKLE WEIGHTS	22					
LONG ARC QUAD - ELASTIC BAND – HAND HELD	23					
LONG ARC QUAD - ELASTIC BAND	24					

EXERCISE **Lower Extremity - Lying & Seated Strengthening and Range of Motion**	EXERCISE NUMBER	PAGE	REPS	SETS	X DAY	HOLD
HAMSTRING CURLS - PRONE - ASSISTED	25					
HAMSTRING CURLS - PRONE	26					
HAMSTRING CURLS - - PRONE - WEIGHTS	27					
HAMSTRING CURLS – PRONE - ELASTIC BAND	28					
HAMSTRING CURLS – ELASTIC BAND	29					
HAMSTRING CURLS – ELASTIC BAND - 2	30					
HAMSTRING CURLS ON BALL	31					
HAMSTRING CURLS - SINGLE LEG - EXERCISE BALL	32					
HIP FLEXION ISOMETRIC	33					
HIP FLEXION ISOMETRIC BILATERAL	34					
HIP FLEXION – ISOMETRIC	35					
STRAIGHT LEG RAISE (SLR)	36					
STRAIGHT LEG RAISE (SLR) – ANKLE WEIGHTS	37					
STRAIGHT LEG RAISE (SLR) - ELASTIC BAND	38					
SEATED MARCHING	39					
SEATED MARCHING - ELASTIC BAND	40					
HIP EXTENSION - PRONE	41					
HIP EXTENSION – PRONE – ANKLE WEIGHTS	42					
HIP EXTENSION – PRONE – ELASTIC BAND	43					
HIP EXTENSION – QUADRUPED	44					
HIP ABDUCTION - SUPINE	45					
HIP ABDUCTION - SUPINE – ANKLE WEIGHTS	46					
HIP ABDUCTION – SUPINE - ELASTIC BAND	47					
HIP ABDUCTION / CLAMS– SUPINE - ELASTIC BAND	48					
MODIFIED HIP ABDUCTION – SIDELYING	49					

EXERCISE **Lower Extremity - Lying & Seated Strengthening and Range of Motion**	EXERCISE NUMBER	PAGE	REPS	SETS	X DAY	HOLD
HIP ABDUCTION – SIDELYING	50					
HIP ABDUCTION – SIDELYING - WEIGHTS	51					
HIP ABDUCTION – SIDELYING - ELASTIC BAND	52					
CLAM SHELLS	53					
SIDELYING CLAM - ELASTIC BAND	54					
HIP ABDUCTION - FIRE HYDRANT - QUADRUPED	55					
HIP ABDUCTION - FIRE HYDRANT – QUADRUPED - ELASTIC BAND	56					
HIP ABDUCTION - SEATED - STRAIGHT LEG	57					
HIP ABDUCTION - SEATED - STRAIGHT LEG – ANKLE WEIGHT	58					
HIP ABDUCTION - SINGLE- SEATED	59					
HIP ABDUCTION - SINGLE- SEATED – ELASTIC BAND	60					
HIP ABDUCTION - BILATERAL- SEATED	61					
HIP ABDUCTION - BILATERAL- SEATED - ELASTIC BAND	62					
HIP ADDUCTION SQUEEZE – SUPINE – KNEES BENT	63					
HIP ADDUCTION SQUEEZE – SUPINE – LEGS STRAIGHT	64					
HIP ADDUCTION - SIDELYING	65					
INTERNAL ROTATION - HEEL SQUEEZE - ISOMETRIC	67					
HIP INTERNAL ROTATION - SUPINE	68					
REVERSE CLAMS - SIDELYING	69					
REVERSE CLAMS - SIDELYING - ELASTIC BAND	70					
HIP INTERNAL ROTATION - SEATED	71					
HIP INTERNAL ROTATION - ELASTIC BAND	72					
HIP EXTERNAL ROTATION - SUPINE	73					

EXERCISE **Lower Extremity - Lying & Seated Strengthening and Range of Motion**	EXERCISE NUMBER	PAGE	REPS	SETS	X DAY	HOLD
HIP EXTERNAL ROTATION - ELASTIC BAND	74					
HIP ROTATIONS – BILATERAL - SIDELYING	75					
HIP ROTATION - SEATED - BALL and ELASTIC BAND	76					
PRESS – BILATERAL – ELASTIC BAND	77					
PRESS – SINGLE LEG – ELASTIC BAND	78					
HIP HIKE - STANDING	79					
HIP HIKE – KNEELING	80					
GLUTE SETS - PRONE	81					
GLUTE SET - SUPINE	82					
GLUTE SQUEEZE - SITTING	83					
GLUTE SCULPT (MAX/MEDIUS)	84					

Worksheets

EXERCISE **Upper Extremity Strengthening and Range of Motion**	EXERCISE NUMBER	PAGE	REPS	SETS	X DAY	HOLD
ELBOW FLEXION EXTENSION - SUPINE	1					
ELBOW FLEXION / EXTENSION - GRAVITY ELIMINATED	2					
BICEPS CURLS – ALTERNATING	3					
BICEPS CURL - SELF FIXATION – ELASTIC BAND	4					
SEATED BICEPS CURLS - ALTERNATING	5					
SEATED BICEPS CURLS - BILATERAL	6					
CONCENTRATION CURLS – SITTING	7					
PREACHER CURL ON BALL	8					
BICEPS CURLS	9					
BICEPS CURLS - RADIOBRACHIALIS - HAMMER CURL	10					
BICEPS CURLS - BRACHIALIS	11					
BICEPS CURLS – ROTATE OUTWARD	12					
BICEPS CURLS – ONE ARM - ELASTIC BAND	13					
BICEPS CURLS – BILATERAL - ELASTIC BAND	14					
BICEPS CURLS - RADIOBRACHIALIS - HAMMER CURL – ONE ARM - ELASTIC BAND	15					
BICEPS CURLS - RADIOBRACHIALIS - HAMMER CURL – BILATERAL - ELASTIC BAND	16					
BICEPS CURLS – BRACHIALIS - ONE ARM - ELASTIC BAND	17					
BICEPS CURL – BRACHIALIS – BILATERAL - ELASTIC BAND	18					
TRICEPS - SELF FIXATION - ELASTIC BAND	19					
OVERHEAD TRICEPS - SELF FIXATION –SEATED OR STANDING - ELASTIC BAND	20					
TRICEP EXTENSION – SITTING OR STANDING - WEIGHT	21					
TRICEP EXTENSION – SITTING OR STANDING – BILATERAL - WEIGHT	22					
ELBOW EXTENSION - BALL	23					

EXERCISE **Upper Extremity Strengthening and Range of Motion**	EXERCISE NUMBER	PAGE	REPS	SETS	X DAY	HOLD
ELBOW EXTENSION - SKULL CRUSHER - BALL	24					
TRICEPS - ELASTIC BAND	25					
TRICEPS - BENT OVER	26					
CHAIR DIPS / PUSH UPS	27					
DIPS OFF CHAIR	28					
PENDULUM SHOULDER FORWARD/BACK	29					
PENDULUM SHOULDER – SIDE TO SIDE	30					
PENDULUM SHOULDER CIRCLES	31					
PENDULUMS - SUPINE	32					
ISOMETRIC FLEXION	33					
SHOULDER FLEXION – SIDELYING	34					
FLEXION – SUPINE - SINGLE OR BILATERAL	35					
FLEXION – SUPINE – SINGLE OR BILATERAL - WEIGHT	36					
FLEXION – SUPINE - DOWEL	37					
FLEXION – SUPINE - DOWEL - Weight	38					
FLEXION - SELF FIXATION – ELASTIC BAND	39					
FLEXION – ELASTIC BAND	40					
FLEXION - STANDING - PALMS DOWN / OVERHAND DOWEL	41					
FLEXION - STANDING - PALMS UP / UNDERHAND DOWEL	42					
FLEXION – PALMS FACING INWARD	43					
FLEXION – PALMS DOWN	44					
V RAISE	45					
V RAISE – WEIGHTS	46					
MILITARY PRESS – DOWEL	47					
MILITARY PRESS - FREE WEIGHTS	48					

EXERCISE Upper Extremity Strengthening and Range of Motion	EXERCISE NUMBER	PAGE	REPS	SETS	X DAY	HOLD
ISOMETRIC EXTENSION	49					
PRONE EXTENSION - EXERCISE BALL	50					
SHOULDER EXTENSION - STANDING	51					
SHOULDER EXTENSION - STANDING - WEIGHTS	52					
EXTENSION – STANDING – DOWEL	53					
EXTENSION - SELF FIXATION - ELASTIC BAND	54					
EXTENSION - ELASTIC BAND	55					
EXTENSION - BILATERAL - ELASTIC BAND	56					
INTERNAL ROTATION – ISOMETRIC	57					
INTERNAL ROTATION - ISOMETRIC- ELEVATED	58					
INTERNAL ROTATION - SIDELYING	59					
INTERNAL ROTATION - ELASTIC BAND	60					
INTERNAL / EXTERNAL ROTATION - STANDING – DOWEL	61					
INTERNAL ROTATION – DOWEL	62					
EXTERNAL ROTATION - ISOMETRIC	63					
EXTERNAL ROTATION - ISOMETRIC – ELEVATED	64					
EXTERNAL ROTATION WITH TOWEL - SIDELYING	65					
EXTERNAL ROTATION – 90/90 - WEIGHTS	66					
EXTERNAL ROTATION - BILATERAL - ELASTIC BAND	67					
EXTERNAL ROTATION - ELASTIC BAND	68					
ADDUCTION – ISOMETRIC	69					
ADDUCTION - ELASTIC BAND	70					
ABDUCTION – ISOMETRIC	71					
HORIZONTAL ABDUCTION - DOWEL	72					

EXERCISE **Upper Extremity** **Strengthening and Range of Motion**	EXERCISE NUMBER	PAGE	REPS	SETS	X DAY	HOLD
HORIZONTAL ABDUCTION/ADDUCTTION - SUPINE	73					
HORIZONTAL ABDUCTION/ADDUCTTION - SUPINE -WEIGHT	74					
ABDUCTION - SIDELYING	75					
HORIZONTAL ABDUCTION - SIDELYING	76					
ABDUCTION – WEIGHT	77					
ABDUCTION – ELASTIC BAND	78					
HORIZONTAL ABDUCTION – BILATERAL - ELASTIC BAND	79					
90/90 ABDUCTION - WEIGHT	80					
LATERAL RAISES	81					
LATERAL RAISES – LEAN FORWARD	82					
LATERAL RAISES – LEAN FORWARD - ARM ROTATION	83					
FRONTAL RAISE – WEIGHTS	84					
UPRIGHT ROW – WEIGHTS	85					
UPRIGHT ROW – ELASTIC BAND	86					
SHRUGS	87					
SHRUGS - WEIGHTS	88					
SHOULDER ROLLS	89					
SHOULDER ROLLS - WEIGHTS	90					
SCAPULAR RETRACTIONS - BILATERAL	91					
SCAPULAR RETRACTION – SINGLE ARM	92					
ELASTIC BAND SCAPULAR RETRACTIONS WITH MINI SHOULDER EXTENSIONS	93					
PRONE RETRACTION	94					
SCAPULAR PROTRACTION - SUPINE - BILATERAL	95					
SCAPULAR PROTRACTION - SUPINE - WEIGHT	96					

Worksheets

EXERCISE Upper Extremity Strengthening and Range of Motion	EXERCISE NUMBER	PAGE	REPS	SETS	X DAY	HOLD
SCAPULAR PROTRACTION - SUPINE - ELASTIC BAND	97					
SCAPULAR PROTRACTION / TABLE PLANK	98					
CHEST PRESS – SEATED or STANDING - ELASTIC BAND	99					
CHEST PRESS – BALL, FLOOR or BENCH- WEIGHTS	100					
DOWEL PRESS – STANDING	101					
CHEST PRESS – STANDING or SEATED	102					
BENT OVER ROWS	103					
ROWS – PRONE	104					
ROWS - ELASTIC BAND	105					
WIDE ROWS - ELASTIC BAND	106					
LOW ROW – ELASTIC BAND	107					
HIGH ROW – ELASTIC BAND	108					
FLY'S – FLOOR - WEIGHT	109					
FLY'S – BALL or BENCH – WEIGHT	110					
WALL PUSH UPS	111					
WALL PUSH UP - BALL	112					
WALL PUSH UP - Triceps uneven	113					
WALL PUSH UP - Hands inverted	114					
WALL PUSH UP - Narrow	115					
WALL PUSH UP – Wide	116					
PUSH UPS - BALL	117					
PUSH UP - MODIFIED	118					
PUSH UP	119					
PUSH UP -DIAMOND	120					
PUSH UP – MODIFIED - BOSU - UNSTABLE	121					

EXERCISE Upper Extremity Strengthening and Range of Motion	EXERCISE NUMBER	PAGE	REPS	SETS	X DAY	HOLD
PUSH UP – BOSU - UNSTABLE	122					
PUSH UP – MODIFIED – INVERTED BOSU - UNSTABLE	123					
PUSH UP – INVERTED BOSU - UNSTABLE	124					

EXERCISE	EXERCISE NUMBER	PAGE	REPS	SETS	X DAY	HOLD
Balance / Standing Exercises						
WIDE BOS DECREASING TO NARROW BOS	1					
NARROW BOS	2					
ARM MOVEMENT	3					
TRUNK ROTATION	4					
EYES SHUTS	5					
HEAD TURNS	6					
READING ALOUD	7					
BALANCE PAD	8					
SPLIT STANCE – SEMI TANDEM	9					
SPLIT STANCE - *Progression*	10					
TANDEM- SHARPENED ROMBERG STANCE	11					
TANDEM STANCE - Progression	12					
SINGLE LEG STANCE (SLS)	13					
SINGLE LEG STANCE (SLS) - *Progression*	14					
SLS – LEG FORWARD	15					
SLS – LEG BACKWARDS	16					
SLS – LEG FORWARD / OPPOSITE ARM UP	17					
SLS – LEG BACKWARDS / OPPOSITE ARM UP	18					
SLS - REACH FORWARD	19					
SLS - REACH TWIST	20					
SINGLE LEG TOE TAP	21					
SINGLE LEG STANCE - CLOCKS	22					
BALL ROLLS - HEEL TOE	23					
BALL ROLLS - LATERAL	24					
SQUAT	25					
SIT TO STAND	26					

EXERCISE Balance / Standing Exercises	EXERCISE NUMBER	PAGE	REPS	SETS	X DAY	HOLD
SQUATS – WALL WITH BALL	27					
SQUATS WITH WEIGHTS	28					
MINI SQUAT - UNSTABLE SUPPORT - FOAM PAD	29					
SQUATS - SINGLE LEG	30					
SIDE TO SIDE WEIGHT SHIFT	31					
FORWARD AND BACKWARDS WEIGHT SHIFTS	32					
SPLIT STANCE WEIGHT SHIFT SIDE TO SIDE	33					
SPLIT STANCE WEIGHT SHIFT FORWARD AND BACKWARDS	34					
WALL FALLS - FORWARD - BALANCE DRILL	35					
WALL FALLS - LATERAL - BALANCE DRILL	36					
WALL FALLS - BACKWARDS - BALANCE DRILL	37					
WALL FALLS - SINGLE LEG - FORWARD - BALANCE DRILL	38					
WALL FALLS - SINGLE LEG - LATERAL - BALANCE DRILL	39					
WALL FALLS - SINGLE LEG - MEDIAL - BALANCE DRILL	40					
WALL FALLS - SINGLE LEG - BACKWARDS - BALANCE DRILL	41					
FALL LATERAL - STEP RECOVERY	42					
FALL FORWARD - STEP RECOVERY	43					
FALL BACKWARD - STEP RECOVERY	44					
TOE TAP ABDUCTION	45					
HIP ABDUCTION - STANDING	46					
HIP EXTENSION – STANDING	47					
HIP FLEXION - STANDING – STRAIGHT LEG RAISE	48					
HIP / KNEE FLEXION - SINGLE LEG	49					
STANDING MARCHING	50					

EXERCISE Balance / Standing Exercises	EXERCISE NUMBER	PAGE	REPS	SETS	X DAY	HOLD
HAMSTRING CURL	51					
TOE RAISES	52					
TOE RAISES IR AND ER	53					
ONE LEGGED TOE RAISE	54					
SINGLE LEG BALANCE FORWARD	55					
SINGLE LEG BALANCE LATERAL	56					
SINGLE LEG BALANCE RETRO	57					
SINGLE LEG STANCE RETROLATERAL	58					
SQUAT	59					
SINGLE LEG SQUAT	60					
LUNGE – STATIC	61					
LUNGE FORWARD/BACKWARD	62					
FOUR CORNER MARCHING IN PLACE	63					
FOUR CORNER MARCHING IN PLACE WITH HEAD TURNS	64					
WALKING ON HEELS FORWARD AND BACKWARDS	65					
WALKING ON TOES FORWARD AND BACKWARDS	66					
TANDEM STANCE AND WALK – FORWARD AND BACKWARDS	67					
RUNNING MAN	68					
HOP STICK - FORWARD	69					
HOP STICK - BACKWARDS	70					
MINI LATERAL LUNGE	71					
SIDE STEPPING	72					
HOP STICK - LATERAL	73					
SINGLE LEG DEAD LIFT	74					

EXERCISE Balance / Standing Exercises	EXERCISE NUMBER	PAGE	REPS	SETS	X DAY	HOLD
CONE TAPS - SINGLE LEG STANCE	75					
CONE TAPS - SINGLE LEG STANCE - UNSTABLE	76					
FIGURE 8 AROUND CONES	77					
FIGURE 8 AROUND CONES – FOOT OR HAND TAP	78					
BALANCE DOUBLE LEG STANCE - WIDE	79					
BALANCE DOUBLE LEG STANCE - NARROW	80					
TANDEM STANCE	81					
TANDEM WALK	82					
SINGLE LEG STANCE - ABDUCTION	83					
SINGLE LEG STANCE - ABDUCTION	84					
SINGLE LEG STANCE – FORWARD KICK	85					
SINGLE LEG STANCE – HAMSTRING CURL	86					
SINGLE LEG SQUAT – LEG FORWARD	87					
SINGLE LEG SQUAT – LEG BACKWARDS	88					
TOE TAP OR HEEL PLACEMENT	89					
PULL UP FOOT TOUCHES ON STEP	90					
ALTERNATING SUSTAINED FOOT TOUCHES ON STEP	91					
STEP UP AND OVER	92					
FORWARD SWING THROUGH STEP	93					
SIDE STEPPING - *REPEAT STEPS 89-93 from a side approach.*	94					

Worksheets

EXERCISE Agility/Reactivity/Speed	EXERCISE NUMBER	PAGE	REPS	SETS	X DAY	HOLD
Four Square Drills	1					
Dots	2					
Ladder Drills	3					
Box Drills	4					
Cones	5					
Hurdles	6					

Myofascial Release

Myofascial release (MFR, self-myofascial release) is an alternative medicine therapy that claims to treat skeletal muscle immobility and pain by relaxing contracted muscles, improving blood and lymphatic circulation, and stimulating the stretch reflex in muscles.

Fascia is a thin, tough, elastic type of connective tissue that wraps most structures within the human body, including muscle. Fascia supports and protects these structures. Osteopathic theory proposes that this soft tissue can become restricted due to psychogenic disease, overuse, trauma, infectious agents, or inactivity, often resulting in pain, muscle tension, and corresponding diminished blood flow. (Wikipedia - *https://en.wikipedia.org/wiki/Myofascial_release*)

Possible Benefits of Myofascial Release

- Muscle relaxation
- Improves muscular and joint range of motion
- Reduces muscle soreness and improves tissue recovery
- Encourages the flow of lymph.
- Improves neuromuscular efficiency.
- Reduces adhesions and scar tissue.
- Releases trigger point (sensitivity and pain) – brings in blood flow and nutrient exchange.
- Maintains normal functional muscular length / Provides optimal length-tension relationship.
- Corrects muscle imbalances

USE

- Roll on foam roller or ball until you find the sore spot or trigger point. When you find this point, stop and rest on it or decrease the range to this particular area and hold for 10-20 seconds.
- Apply pressure to muscle area only. Try not to roll over bones, joints or directly on the spine (you can use a ball over the muscles on the side of the spine).
- Use this as a part of your warmup for particular areas you are exercising that day (for instance the hamstrings, calves and quadricep on leg strengthening day)
- You can use this technique on additional days for trouble areas and can even devote a dedicated session for whole body myofascial release.

Equipment Needed: FOAM ROLLER and/or TEXTURED or SOFT MASSAGE BALL

EXERCISE Myofascial Release	EXERCISE NUMBER	NOTES
ANTERIOR CHEST - BALL	1	
ANTERIOR CHEST - FOAM ROLL	2	
LATISSIMUS DORSI – BALL	3	
LATISSIMUS DORSI - FOAM ROLL	4	
TRICEP – FOAM ROLL	5	
OCCIPITAL RELEASE - FOAM ROLL	6	
THORACIC MOBILIZATION – SUPINE - FOAM ROLL	7	
THORACIC MOBILIZATION – STANDING - FOAM ROLL	8	
LUMBAR – STANDING – BALL - can do with foam roll	9	
LUMBAR – SUPINE – FOAM ROLLER	10	
HIP FLEXORS - BALL	11	
HIP FLEXORS – FOAM ROLL	12	
QUADRICEPS – BILATERAL - FOAM ROLL	13	
QUADRICEP – SINGLE - FOAM ROLL	14	
GLUTE /PIRIFORMIS - FOAM ROLL	15	
HIP ADDUCTORS – FOAM ROLL	16	
HAMSTRING – BILATERAL - FOAM ROLL	17	
HAMSTRING – SINGLE – FOAM ROLL	18	
CALVES – BILATERAL - FOAM ROLL	19	
CALVES – SINGLE - FOAM ROLL	20	
ILIOTIBIAL BAND (IT Band) - FOAM ROLL	21	
ILIOTIBIAL BAND (IT Band) - BALL	22	
PLANTAR FASCIA ROLLING – BALL	23	
PLANTAR FASCIA ROLLING - COLD SODA CAN	24	

Myofascial Release

	_____ Reps _____ Sets _____X Day _____Hold		_____ Reps _____ Sets _____X Day _____Hold
1	Notes:	**2**	Notes:

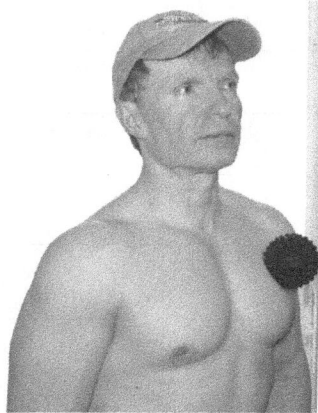

ANTERIOR CHEST - BALL

Face towards the wall and place small ball at the outside of chest. Bend knees up and down to find the target point and hold.

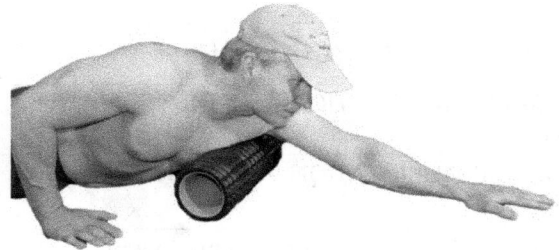

ANTERIOR CHEST - FOAM ROLL

Lie face down so that a foam roll is under the upper part of your arm and chest. Using your other arm and legs, roll forward and back across this area.

	_____ Reps _____ Sets _____X Day _____Hold		_____ Reps _____ Sets _____X Day _____Hold
3	Notes:	**4**	Notes:

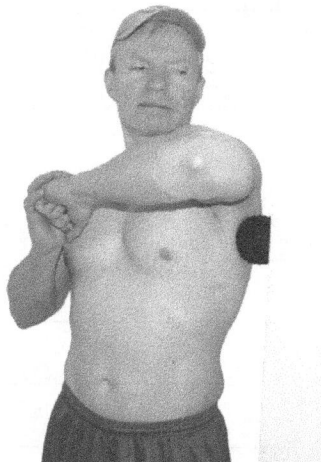

LATISSIMUS DORSI – BALL

Turn with your target side towards the wall and place small ball on the side under the shoulder. Bend knees up and down to find the target point and hold.

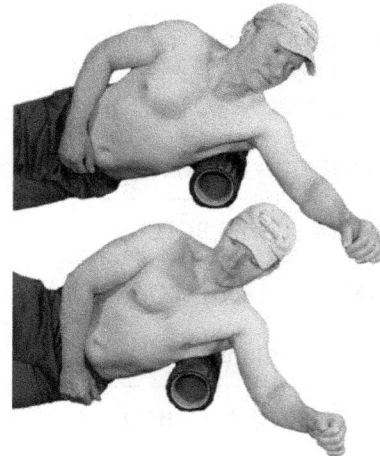

LATISSIMUS DORSI - FOAM ROLL

Lie on your side so that a foam roll is under the upper part of your arm and back. Using your other arm and legs, roll forward and back across this area.

_____ Reps _____ Sets _____ X Day _____ Hold	_____ Reps _____ Sets _____ X Day _____ Hold

5 Notes:

6 Notes:

TRICEP – FOAM ROLL

In a sidelying position, place your tricep on the foam roll. Use the opposite arm and your body to help roll out the arm on the foam roll.

OCCIPITAL RELEASE - FOAM ROLL

Lie on your back and put a foam roll under the back of your head. Turn your head slowly from side to side.

_____ Reps _____ Sets _____ X Day _____ Hold	_____ Reps _____ Sets _____ X Day _____ Hold

7 Notes:

8 Notes:

THORACIC MOBILIZATION – SUPINE - FOAM ROLL

Lie on a foam roller. While supporting your neck, roll up and down your mid-back.

THORACIC MOBILIZATION – STANDING - FOAM ROLL

Stand with a foam roll behind your upper back. Slowly perform mini-squats and allow the foam roller to roll up and down your back for a self-massage.

	_____ Reps _____ Sets _____X Day _____Hold
9	Notes:

LUMBAR – STANDING – BALL - can do with foam roll

Place small ball in lower back on the side of the spine. DO NOT roll directly over the spine. Slowly perform mini-squats and allow the ball to roll up and down your back for a self-massage.
*Can use foam roll behind lower back and follow above directions.

	_____ Reps _____ Sets _____X Day _____Hold
10	Notes:

LUMBAR – SUPINE – FOAM ROLLER

Lie on a foam roll under the lower back. While supporting your upper body, roll up and down your lower back.

	_____ Reps _____ Sets _____X Day _____Hold
11	Notes:

Ball under hip flexor

HIP FLEXORS - BALL

Lie on your stomach and place small ball under hip flexor. Roll up and down ball making small movements and hold on the target muscle.

	_____ Reps _____ Sets _____X Day _____Hold
12	Notes:

HIP FLEXORS – FOAM ROLL

Lie on your stomach and place foam roll under both hip flexors. Roll up and down avoiding rolling directly over hip bones.

	_____ Reps _____ Sets _____ X Day _____ Hold		_____ Reps _____ Sets _____ X Day _____ Hold
13	Notes:	14	Notes:

QUADRICEPS – BILATERAL - FOAM ROLL

Lie face down so that a foam roll is under the top of your thighs. Using your arms propped on your elbows, roll forward and back across this area.

QUADRICEP – SINGLE - FOAM ROLL

Lie face down so that a foam roll is under the top of your target thigh. Cross your other leg over the top of your target leg. Using your arms propped on your elbows, roll forward and back across this area.

	_____ Reps _____ Sets _____ X Day _____ Hold		_____ Reps _____ Sets _____ X Day _____ Hold
15	Notes:	16	Notes:

GLUTE /PIRIFORMIS - FOAM ROLL

Sit on a foam roll and cross your affected leg on top of your other knee. Lean slightly towards your target side. Using your arms and unaffected leg roll forward and back across your buttock area.

HIP ADDUCTORS – FOAM ROLL

Lie on your stomach supported by arms and lace your inner thigh on the roller. Roll and compress the target thigh muscle.

	_____ Reps _____ Sets _____X Day _____Hold
17	Notes:

HAMSTRING – BILATERAL - FOAM ROLL

Sit on a foam roll under both thighs. Using your arms, roll forward and back across this area

	_____ Reps _____ Sets _____X Day _____Hold
18	Notes:

HAMSTRING – SINGLE – FOAM ROLL

Sit on a foam roll under thigh. Using your arms, roll forward and back across this area.

	_____ Reps _____ Sets _____X Day _____Hold
19	Notes:

CALVES – BILATERAL - FOAM ROLL

Sit with the foam roll under your both your calves. Lift your body up with your arms and roll forward and back across your calf area. Try turning toes in and out to access the inside and outside of calf areas. Do not roll in the crease of your knee.

	_____ Reps _____ Sets _____X Day _____Hold
20	Notes: -

CALVES – SINGLE - FOAM ROLL

Sit with the foam roll under your target calf and cross your other leg on top. Lift your body up with your arms and roll forward and back across your calf area. Do not roll in the crease of your knee.

_____ Reps _____ Sets _____X Day _____Hold		_____ Reps _____ Sets _____X Day _____Hold
21	**Notes:**	**22**

ILIOTIBIAL BAND (IT Band) - FOAM ROLL

Lie on your side with a foam roll under your bottom thigh. Use your arms and unaffected leg and then roll up and down the foam roll along the outside of your thigh.

ILIOTIBIAL BAND (IT Band) - BALL

Lie on your side or sit in chair. Hold small ball and move along the outside of the thigh. Hold on the target muscle.

_____ Reps _____ Sets _____X Day _____Hold		_____ Reps _____ Sets _____X Day _____Hold
23	**Notes:**	**24**

PLANTAR FASCIA ROLLING – BALL

Sit and place ball under foot. Roll plantar fascia over ball back and forth.

PLANTAR FASCIA ROLLING - COLD SODA CAN

Sit and place cold soda can under foot. Roll plantar fascia over can back and forth.

Flexibility (Stretching)

Range of motion within a joint across various planes of motion that can be increased with stretching. This is needed to prevent decreased range of motion in a joint. Joint mobility can be inhibited by body habitués, genetics, connective tissue elasticity, skin that surrounds the joint, or the joint itself.

Some of the benefits of stretching: *(ACE Personal Training Manual)*	• Increased physical efficiency and performance. • Decreased risk of injury by decreasing resistance in various tissues. • Increased blood supply and nutrients to joint structures. • Improved nutrient exchange by increasing the quantity and decreasing the thickness of synovial fluid in the joint. • Increased neuromuscular coordination. • Improved muscular balance and postural awareness. • Reduced muscular tension. *(Bryant & Daniel, Ace Personal Training Manual, 2003, pg 306-307)*
Things to remember when stretching	• It is always better to stretch a warm muscle (*see Warm up and Cool down*) when the tissue temperature is above normal. Think of putting an elastic band in the freezer compared to heating it before stretching. Which do you think will get a better stretch? • Static stretching is best for the type for beginning athletes. Static stretching is a slow, gradual lengthening of the connective tissue (tendon, muscles and ligaments) through a full range of motion to the point of discomfort – not pain. This stretch should be held for at least 30 seconds, but no longer than two minutes. • Dynamic stretching consists of controlled leg and arm swings that take you to the limits of your range of motion. This type of stretching is appropriate to perform part of a warmup and/or cool down. • Ballistic stretching is a rapid, bouncing movement that may be appropriate in some sports. The problem is that there is also a high-risk factor for injury and should only be done with a professional's guidance. • Again, always remember to warm up before stretching. Repeat all stretches 2-3 times and hold for 15-30 seconds up to 60 seconds) unless otherwise indicated. • Some evidence shows that static stretching may be more beneficial at the end of the exercise program when there is more certainty that the muscles have warmed up. • Dynamic stretching may be more beneficial at the beginning of the exercise program as part of your warmup. This can also be done at the end as part of the cool down.

EXERCISE Flexibility (Stretching)	EXERCISE NUMBER	NOTES
INVERSION	1	
EVERSION	2	
ANTERIOR TIBIALIS	3	
PLANTARFLEXION	4	
DORSIFLEXION - STRAP	5	
DORSIFLEXION - FLOOR ASSISTED	6	
STANDING CALF STRETCH - GASTROC	7	
STANDING CALF STRETCH - GASTROC – HAND ON KNEE	8	
GASTROCNEMIUS STAIR STRETCH	9	
STANDING CALF STRETCH - SOLEUS	10	
HAMSTRING STRETCH – TOWEL, BAND, STRAP or BELT	11	
HAMSTRING STRETCH – TOWEL, BAND, STRAP or BELT	12	
HAMSTRING STRETCH - TABLE, BED OR COUCH	13	
HAMSTRING / KNEE EXTENSION STRETCH - SEATED	14	
HAMSTRING STRETCH - STANDING	15	
TOE TOUCH – STANDING - NARROW or WIDE BOS	16	
HEEL SLIDES - SELF ASSISTED	17	
HEEL SLIDES - LONG SIT ASSISTED - TOWEL, BAND, STRAP or BELT	18	
HEEL SLIDES - SUPINE	19	
KNEE BENDS - EXERCISE BALL	20	
KNEE FLEXION – SELF ASSISTED - PRONE	21	
KNEE FLEXION – BELT ASSISTED - PRONE	22	
HEEL SLIDES - SELF ASSISTED	23	
HEEL SLIDES - SEATED	24	
KNEE FLEXION – SCOOT FORWARD - SEATED	25	

EXERCISE Flexibility (Stretching)	EXERCISE NUMBER	NOTES
KNEE FLEXION – STAIR OR STEP	26	
PIRIFORMIS STRETCH	27	
PIRIFORMIS STRETCH - EXERCISE BALL	28	
PIRIFORMIS STRETCH - LONG SIT	29	
PIRIFORMIS STRETCH – STANDING	30	
HIP FLEXOR STRETCH - SIDE OF BALL or CHAIR	31	
HIP FLEXOR STRETCH - STANDING	32	
HIP FLEXOR STRETCH - HALF KNEEL	33	
RUNNER'S STRETCH - MODIFIED	34	
HIP FLEXOR STRETCH – SUPINE	35	
HIP FLEXOR STRETCH – SUPINE - 2	36	
QUAD STRETCH - SIDELYING	37	
QUAD STRETCH - STANDING	38	
KNEE FALL OUT STRETCH or FROG STRETCH	39	
BUTTERFLY STRETCH	40	
HIP ADDUCTOR STRECH – KNEELING	41	
HIP ADDUCTOR STRECH - STANDING	42	
HIP EXTERNAL ROTATION STRETCH - SUPINE	43	
HIP INTERNAL ROTATION STRETCH - SEATED	44	
IT BAND STRETCH - STANDING	45	
IT BAND STRETCH -- SIDELYING	46	
NECK ROTATION and SIDE BENDS	47	
NECK FLEXION AND EXTENSION	48	
TRUNK FLEXION - SEATED	49	
LOW BACK STRETCH - SEATED	50	
LOW BACK STRETCH – STANDING - STRAIGHT & LATERAL	51	
LOW BACK STRETCH – RAIL OR DOORKNOB	52	

EXERCISE Flexibility (Stretching)	EXERCISE NUMBER	NOTES
PRAYER STRETCH and LATERAL	53	
PRAYER STRETCH - EXERCISE BALL	54	
CAT AND CAMEL	55	
KNEE TO CHEST STRETCH - SINGLE and BILATERAL	56	
PRONE ON ELBOWS	57	
PRESS UPS	58	
TRUNK ROTATION STRETCH – SINGLE LEG	59	
LOWER TRUNK ROTATIONS – BILATERAL	60	
TRUNK ROTATION - SEATED	61	
TRUNK ROTATION - STANDING or SEATED – DOWEL	62	
LATERAL TRUNK STRETCH - SINGLE, SEATED or STANDING	63	
LATERAL TRUNK STRETCH - BILATERAL SEATED or STANDING	64	
FLEXION - SUPINE - DOWEL	65	
WALL WALK	66	
FLEXION - TABLE SLIDE	67	
FLEXION - TABLE SLIDE - BALL	68	
EXTERNAL ROTATION - SUPINE – DOWEL *INTERNAL ROTATION ON OPPOSITE ARM*	69	
EXTERNAL ROTATION - 90-90 - DOWEL	70	
EXTERNAL ROTATION – SEATED – DOWEL *INTERNAL ROTATION ON OPPOSITE ARM*	71	
EXTERNAL ROTATION – STANDING – DOWEL *INTERNAL ROTATION ON OPPOSITE ARM*	72	
ABDUCTION - TABLE SLIDE - BALL	75	
ABDUCTION WITH DOWEL	76	
LYING DOWN EXTENSION - TABLE or BED	77	
WAND EXTENSION - STANDING	78	
CHEST STRETCH – SEATED, STANDING, or SUPINE	79	

Flexibility (Stretching)

EXERCISE Flexibility (Stretching)	EXERCISE NUMBER	NOTES
TRICEP STRETCH - STRAP or TOWEL	82	
POSTERIOR SHOULDER/DELTOID RELEASE	83	
POSTERIOR CAPSULE STRETCH	84	

Stretching / Range of Motion (ROM)

Inversion

	_____ Reps _____ Sets _____X Day _____Hold
1	**Notes:**

INVERSION

Sit and cross your legs so that the target leg is on top. Hold your foot and pull upwards until a stretch is felt along the side of your ankle.

Eversion

	_____ Reps _____ Sets _____X Day _____Hold
2	**Notes:**

EVERSION

Sit and cross your legs so that the target leg is on top. Hold your foot and push downward until a stretch is felt along the inner side of your ankle.

Anterior Tibialis (Ant Tib)

	_____ Reps _____ Sets _____X Day _____Hold
3	**Notes:**

ANTERIOR TIBIALIS

Kneel upright and slowly sit back onto legs forcing heels down towards floor. Sit back until stretch is felt.

Plantarflexion (PF) _DF not shown_

	_____ Reps _____ Sets _____X Day _____Hold
4	**Notes:**

PLANTARFLEXION

Sit and place your affected foot on a firm surface. Use one hand bend the ankle downward as shown.

DORSIFLEXION – _Not shown_
Sit and place your affected foot on a firm surface. Use one hand under foot to push up towards shin (see #5 for movement)

Dorsiflexion (DF)

	_____ Reps _____ Sets _____ X Day _____ Hold		_____ Reps _____ Sets _____ X Day _____ Hold
5	Notes:	**6**	Notes:

DORSIFLEXION - STRAP

Sit with heel on floor and leg straight. Place belt/strap on forefoot and pull back until stretch is felt.

DORSIFLEXION - FLOOR ASSISTED

Sit and slide your foot back towards under the chair until a stretch is felt at the ankle.

Gastroc/Soleus

	_____ Reps _____ Sets _____ X Day _____ Hold		_____ Reps _____ Sets _____ X Day _____ Hold
7	Notes:	**8**	Notes:

Target Leg

STANDING CALF STRETCH - GASTROC

Stand in front of a wall, chair, or other sturdy object. Step forward with one foot and maintain your toes on both feet to be pointed straight forward. Keep the leg behind you with a straight knee during the stretch. Lean forward as you allow your front knee to bend until a stretch is felt along the back of your leg. Move closer or further away from the wall to control the stretch of the back leg.

Target Leg

STANDING CALF STRETCH - GASTROC – HAND ON KNEE

Step forward with one foot and place hand on thigh. Maintain your toes on both feet to be pointed straight forward. Keep the leg behind you with a straight knee during the stretch. Lean forward as you allow your front knee to bend until a stretch is felt along the back of your leg. You can adjust the bend of the front knee to control the stretch.

Flexibility (Stretching)

	_____ Reps _____ Sets _____ X Day _____ Hold		_____ Reps _____ Sets _____ X Day _____ Hold
9	Notes:	10	Notes:

GASTROCNEMIUS STAIR STRETCH

Stand with the middle of your foot on the edge of the stairs while holding onto the railing. Slowly drop heels off until you feel a stretch in the back of your legs keeping your knees straight.

STANDING CALF STRETCH - SOLEUS

Stand in front of a wall, chair or other sturdy object. Step forward with one foot and maintain your toes on both feet to be pointed straight forward. Keep the leg behind you with a slightly bent knee during the stretch. Lean forward towards the wall and support yourself with your arms as you allow your front knee to bend until a gentle stretch is felt along the back of your leg. *Move closer or further away from the wall to control the stretch of the back leg. You can also adjust the bend of the front knee to control the stretch.

Hamstring / Knee Extension

	_____ Reps _____ Sets _____ X Day _____ Hold		_____ Reps _____ Sets _____ X Day _____ Hold
11	Notes:	12	Notes:

HAMSTRING STRETCH – TOWEL, BAND, STRAP or BELT

Lie down on your back and hook a towel/strap under your foot and draw up your leg until a stretch is felt under your leg/calf area. Keep your knee in a straightened position during the stretch. To increase stretch move strap to forefoot and flex foot.

HAMSTRING STRETCH – TOWEL, BAND, STRAP or BELT

While pushing down on thigh above knee cap with opposite hand, pull on towel/ strap to lift heel from floor. Keep thigh flat. To increase stretch move strap to forefoot and flex foot and/or lean forward at the hip.

_____ Reps _____ Sets _____ X Day _____ Hold

13	Notes:

HAMSTRING STRETCH - TABLE, BED OR COUCH

Sit on a raised flat surface where you can prop your target leg up on it such as a treatment table, couch or bed. While keeping your knee straight, slowly lean forward and reach your hands towards your foot until a gentle stretch is felt along the back of your knee/thigh. Hold and then return to starting position and repeat. Allow gravity to stretch your knee towards a more straightened position.
* Can use strap, towel or belt around forefoot as in #12

_____ Reps _____ Sets _____ X Day _____ Hold

14	Notes:

HAMSTRING / KNEE EXTENSION STRETCH - SEATED

Sit and tighten your top thigh muscle to press the back of your knee downward towards the ground. You should feel a gentle stretch in the back of your knee.

* To increase stretch put strap to forefoot, flex foot and lean forward at the hip.

_____ Reps _____ Sets _____ X Day _____ Hold

15	Notes:

HAMSTRING STRETCH - STANDING

Stand and rest your foot on a stool/box/step with your knee straight. Gently lean forward at the hips until a stretch is felt behind your knee/thigh. Keep your back straight. *To increase stretch, flex your foot at the ankle, and/or put strap to forefoot and flex foot. If on stair, you can put foot on 2nd or 3rd step.

_____ Reps _____ Sets _____ X Day _____ Hold

16	Notes:

TOE TOUCH – STANDING - NARROW or WIDE BOS

Stand and bend forward at waist keep legs straight and reach for toes. Can perform with either narrow or wide base of support.

Knee Flexion

	_____Reps _____Sets _____X Day _____Hold		_____Reps _____Sets _____X Day _____Hold
17	**Notes:**	**18**	**Notes:**

HEEL SLIDES - SELF ASSISTED

Lie on your back with knees straight and slide the target heel towards your buttock as you bend your knee. Use the unaffected leg to assist the bending. Hold a gentle stretch in this position and then return to original position.

HEEL SLIDES - LONG SIT ASSISTED - TOWEL, BAND, STRAP or BELT

Sit with legs straight. Can place a small hand towel under your heel to help slide. Loop a band around your foot and pull your knee into a bend position as your foot slides towards your buttock. Hold a gentle stretch and then return back to original position.

	_____Reps _____Sets _____X Day _____Hold		_____Reps _____Sets _____X Day _____Hold
19	**Notes:**	**20**	**Notes:**

HEEL SLIDES - SUPINE

Lie on your back with knees straight and slide the target heel towards your buttock as you bend your knee. Hold a gentle stretch in this position and then return to original position.

KNEE BENDS - EXERCISE BALL

Lie on your back and place your heels on an exercise ball. Roll it closer to your buttocks as your knees and hips bend as shown. Hold and then return to original position. *If you have limited range in one knee, use the other leg to help increase range of motion.

_____ Reps _____ Sets _____X Day _____Hold		_____ Reps _____ Sets _____X Day _____Hold
21	Notes:	**22**	Notes:

KNEE FLEXION – SELF ASSISTED - PRONE

Lie face down and bend your target knee with the assistance of your unaffected leg.

KNEE FLEXION – BELT ASSISTED - PRONE

Lie face down with a strap looped around your target side ankle or foot. Use the belt to pull the knee into a bent position allowing for a stretch.

_____ Reps _____ Sets _____X Day _____Hold		_____ Reps _____ Sets _____X Day _____Hold
23	Notes:	**24**	Notes:

HEEL SLIDES - SELF ASSISTED

It and slide your heel towards your buttock with the assist of the unaffected leg. Hold a gentle stretch and then return foot forward to original position.

HEEL SLIDES - SEATED – can use towel or paper under foot to help slide

Sit and place your feet on the floor (can put target foot on a towel or paper to help slide if needed). Slowly slide your foot closer towards you. Hold a gentle stretch and then return foot forward to original position.

	_____ Reps _____ Sets _____X Day _____Hold
25	**Notes:**

Plant foot. Scoot hips forward.

KNEE FLEXION – SCOOT FORWARD - SEATED

Sit and slide your foot back to a bent knee position. Keep your foot planted on the ground and scoot forward until a stretch is felt at the knee. Hold the stretch and then scoot back to original position.

	_____ Reps _____ Sets _____X Day _____Hold
26	**Notes:**

KNEE FLEXION – STAIR OR STEP

Place target foot on stool or step with bent knee. Gently bend forward keeping heel on step. Hold the stretch and then return to original position.

Piriformis

	_____ Reps _____ Sets _____X Day _____Hold
27	**Notes:**

PIRIFORMIS STRETCH

Lie on your back with both knees bent. Cross your target leg on the other knee. Hold your unaffected thigh and pull it up towards your chest until a stretch is felt in the buttock.

	_____ Reps _____ Sets _____X Day _____Hold
28	**Notes:**

PIRIFORMIS STRETCH - EXERCISE BALL

Lie on your back with one foot placed on the ball. Cross your other leg over the knee of the leg on the ball and gently roll the ball back towards your chest until a stretch is felt in the buttock.

	_____ Reps _____ Sets _____X Day _____Hold
29	**Notes:**

PIRIFORMIS STRETCH - LONG SIT

Sit with one knee straight and the other bent and placed over the opposite knee. Gentle turn your body towards the bend knee side.

	_____ Reps _____ Sets _____X Day _____Hold
30	**Notes:**

PIRIFORMIS STRETCH – STANDING

Stand with unaffected leg crossed in front of target side. Lean forward reaching for foot on target side until stretch is felt in the buttock.

Hip Flexors

	_____ Reps _____ Sets _____X Day _____Hold
31	**Notes:**

HIP FLEXOR STRETCH - SIDE OF BALL or CHAIR

Sit on edge of chair or ball. Bend your front knee (unaffected side) and lean forward until a stretch is felt along the front of the target hip.

	_____ Reps _____ Sets _____X Day _____Hold
32	**Notes:**

HIP FLEXOR STRETCH - STANDING

Stand and bend one knee forward (unaffected side) and the other in back. Stand up straight leaning slightly backward until a stretch is felt along the front of the target hip.

_____ Reps _____ Sets _____X Day _____Hold		_____ Reps _____ Sets _____X Day _____Hold
33	**Notes:**	**34** **Notes:**

HIP FLEXOR STRETCH - HALF KNEEL – with or without pad under knee

Begin in a half-kneeling position (you may want to use a pad or pillow for cushion). Bend your front knee (unaffected side) and lean forward until a stretch is felt along the front of the target hip.

RUNNER'S STRETCH - MODIFIED

Stretch target leg in back and bend other knee in front. Bend your front knee (unaffected side) and lean forward until a stretch is felt along the front of the target hip.

_____ Reps _____ Sets _____X Day _____Hold		_____ Reps _____ Sets _____X Day _____Hold
35	**Notes:**	**36** **Notes:**

HIP FLEXOR STRETCH – SUPINE

Lie on a table, high bed or matt and let the affected leg lower towards the floor until a stretch is felt along the front of your thigh.

HIP FLEXOR STRETCH – SUPINE

Lie on a table, high bed or matt and let the affected leg lower towards the floor until a stretch is felt along the front of your thigh. At the same time, grasp your opposite knee and pull it towards your chest.

Quadriceps (Quad)

	_____ Reps _____ Sets _____ X Day _____ Hold		_____ Reps _____ Sets _____ X Day _____ Hold
37	**Notes:**	**38**	**Notes:**

QUAD STRETCH - SIDELYING

Lie on your side and reach back holding the top of your foot with bent knee until a stretch is felt.

QUAD STRETCH - STANDING

Stand straight up and bend your knee in back holding your ankle/foot. Gently pull your knee/thigh back in alignment with the standing leg.

Adductor

	_____ Reps _____ Sets _____ X Day _____ Hold		_____ Reps _____ Sets _____ X Day _____ Hold
39	**Notes:**	**40**	**Notes:**

One Leg

Both Legs

KNEE FALL OUT STRETCH or FROG STRETCH

Lie on your back with one knee bent. Slowly lower your knee to the side as you stretch the inner thigh/hip area. Frog Stretch: Let both knees fall to the side at the same time.

BUTTERFLY STRETCH

Sit on the floor or mat and bend your knees placing the bottom of your feet together. Slowly let your knees lower towards the floor until a stretch is felt at your inner thighs.

_____ Reps _____ Sets _____ X Day _____ Hold	_____ Reps _____ Sets _____ X Day _____ Hold
41 Notes:	**42** Notes:

Target Leg

HIP ADDUCTOR STRECH – KNEELING

Kneel down on your target side knee. Place the opposite leg directly out to the side. Lean towards the side as you bend the knee for a stretch to the inner thigh of the target leg.

Target Leg

HIP ADDUCTOR STRECH - STANDING

Stand with feet spread wide apart. Slowly bend your knee to allow for a gentle stretch of the opposite leg. Maintain a straight knee on the target leg the entire time. You should feel a stretch on the inner thigh.

External Rotation / Internal Rotation

_____ Reps _____ Sets _____ X Day _____ Hold	_____ Reps _____ Sets _____ X Day _____ Hold
43 Notes:	**44** Notes:

HIP EXTERNAL ROTATION STRETCH - SUPINE

Lie on your back with your leg crossed over your knee. Use your hand and push the crossed knee away from you.

HIP INTERNAL ROTATION STRETCH - SEATED

Sit on a chair with your legs spread apart and feet planted on the ground. Use your hand to draw your knee inward as shown.

Iliotibial Band (IT Band)

	_____ Reps _____ Sets _____ X Day _____ Hold
45	**Notes:**

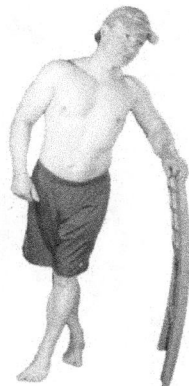

IT BAND STRETCH - STANDING

Stand and cross the target leg behind your unaffected leg. Lean forward and towards the unaffected side while using your arm for balance support.

	_____ Reps _____ Sets _____ X Day _____ Hold
46	**Notes:**

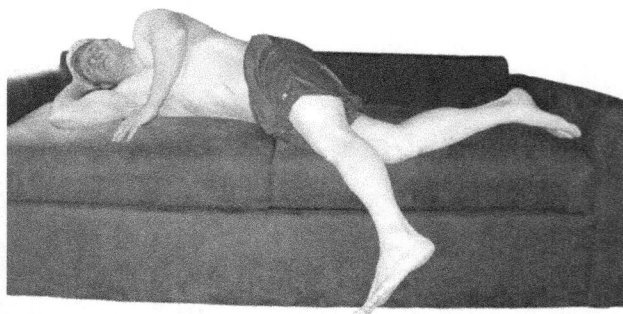

IT BAND STRETCH -- SIDELYING

Lie on bed or couch on unaffected side with target side towards ceiling. Bend lower leg for support. Allow upper leg to drop over side of bed. Keep knee straight and point toe towards floor. May need to roll upper hip backwards in order to feel stretch on side of hip/thigh/knee.

NECK

	_____ Reps _____ Sets _____ X Day _____ Hold
47	**Notes:**

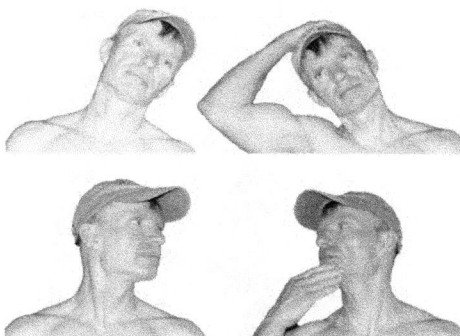

NECK ROTATION and SIDE BENDS

SIDE BENDS: (_Top_) Tilt your head as if you are trying to touch your ear to your shoulder. For extra stretch gently use your hand to increase range and hold.
ROTATION: (_Bottom_) Turn your head to the side as if looking over your shoulder. For an extra stretch gently use your hand on your chin to increase range and hold.

	_____ Reps _____ Sets _____ X Day _____ Hold
48	**Notes:**

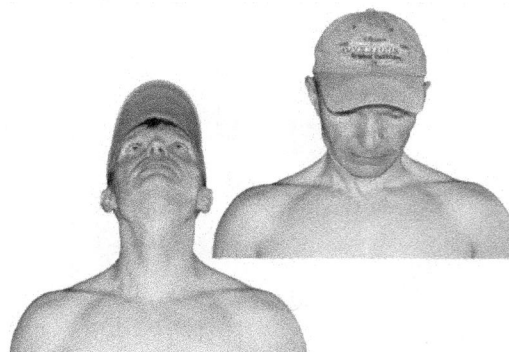

NECK FLEXION AND EXTENSION

EXTENSION: Look up as if you are looking at the sky moving your neck only.
FLEXION: Look down as if you are looking at the floor. For an extra stretch gently put both hands behind your head to move chin towards the chest and hold.

BACK

	_____ Reps _____ Sets _____X Day _____Hold	
49	**Notes:**	

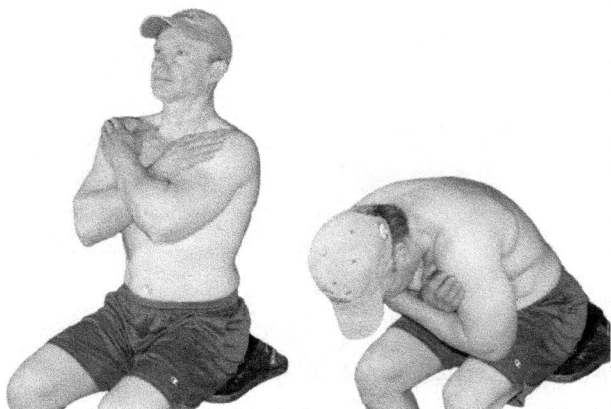

TRUNK FLEXION - SEATED

Sit and cross your arms over your chest. Slowly curl your back forward in order to round your upper back.

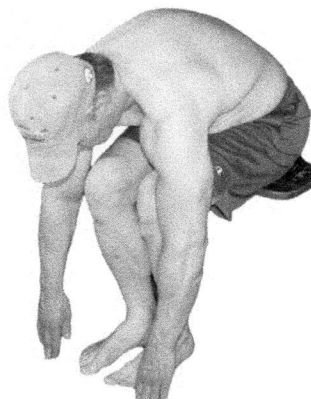

	_____ Reps _____ Sets _____X Day _____Hold	
50	**Notes:**	

LOW BACK STRETCH - SEATED

Sit and slowly bend forward reaching your hands for the floor. Bend your trunk and head forward and down.

	_____ Reps _____ Sets _____X Day _____Hold	
51	**Notes:**	

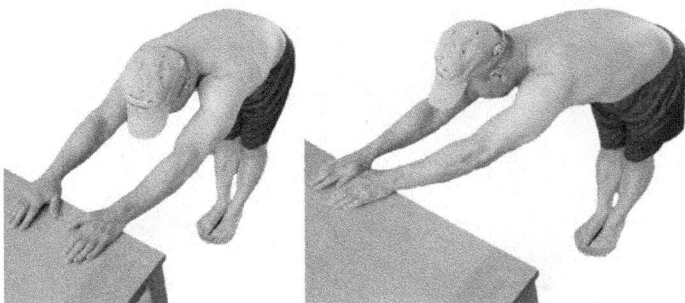

LOW BACK STRETCH – STANDING - STRAIGHT & LATERAL

Stand in front of a table / chair or other surface and bend forward at the waist. Support yourself with your hands on a surface.

Reach to the side for a lateral bend (see #53)

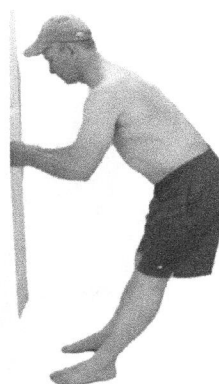

	_____ Reps _____ Sets _____X Day _____Hold	
52	**Notes:**	

LOW BACK STRETCH – RAIL OR DOORKNOB

Hold onto doorknob, rail or other unmovable surface and pull while moving hips back and hold.

	_____ Reps _____ Sets _____ X Day _____ Hold
53	**Notes:**

Lateral

Straight

PRAYER STRETCH and LATERAL

STRAIGHT: Start on your hands and knees. Slowly lower your buttocks towards your feet until a stretch is felt along your back and or buttocks.

LATERAL: Start on your hands and knees. Slowly lower your buttocks towards your feet. Lower your chest towards the floor as you reach out towards the side.

	_____ Reps _____ Sets _____ X Day _____ Hold
54	**Notes:**

PRAYER STRETCH - EXERCISE BALL

Kneel with an exercise ball in front of you. Slowly lean forward and roll the ball forward until a stretch is felt.

*Can do lateral movement as in #53

	_____ Reps _____ Sets _____ X Day _____ Hold
55	**Notes:**

CAT AND CAMEL

Start on your hands and knees. Raise up your back and arch it towards the ceiling (cat). Return to a lowered position and arch your back the opposite direction (camel).

	_____ Reps _____ Sets _____ X Day _____ Hold
56	**Notes:**

Both Legs

One Leg

KNEE TO CHEST STRETCH - SINGLE and BILATERAL

BILATERAL: Lie on your back and hold your knees while pulling up towards your chest and hold.
SINGLE: Lie on your back and hold your knee while pulling up towards your chest and hold. Opposite leg can be straight or bent.

Trunk Extension

	_____ Reps _____ Sets _____ X Day _____ Hold		_____ Reps _____ Sets _____ X Day _____ Hold
57	Notes:	58	Notes:

PRONE ON ELBOWS

Lie on your stomach. Slowly press up and prop yourself up on your elbows. Keep hips on floor/mat.

PRESS UPS

Lie on your stomach. Slowly press up and arch your back using your arms. Keep hips on floor/mat.

Trunk Rotation

	_____ Reps _____ Sets _____ X Day _____ Hold		_____ Reps _____ Sets _____ X Day _____ Hold
59	Notes:	60	Notes:

TRUNK ROTATION STRETCH – SINGLE LEG

Lie on your back with arms to the sides. Bend one knee and then raise it up and across your body. Allow your trunk to rotate for a gentle stretch to the spine. Hold and then repeat.

LOWER TRUNK ROTATIONS – BILATERAL

Lie on your back with your knees bent and gently move your knees side-to-side.

_____ Reps _____ Sets _____ X Day _____ Hold		_____ Reps _____ Sets _____ X Day _____ Hold	
61	Notes:	**62**	Notes:

TRUNK ROTATION - SEATED

Sit up as tall with erect posture. Rotate in one direction, using your hand to press against the opposite thigh to aide in further rotation. Exhale to increase the rotation and stretch. Return to the starting position, maintain an upright posture -repeat in the opposite direction.

TRUNK ROTATION - STANDING or SEATED – DOWEL

Stand or sit holding dowel in hands. Slowly rotate trunk in one direction and then in the opposite direction.

Lateral

_____ Reps _____ Sets _____ X Day _____ Hold		_____ Reps _____ Sets _____ X Day _____ Hold	
63	Notes:	**64**	Notes:

LATERAL TRUNK STRETCH - SINGLE SEATED or STANDING

Raise your arm and bend to the opposite side for a stretch. Hold and repeat with opposite arm.

LATERAL TRUNK STRETCH - BILATERAL SEATED or STANDING

Clasp hands together and raise arms over head. Bend to one side. Hold and repeat in opposite direction.

Shoulder Flexion

_____ Reps _____ Sets _____ X Day _____ Hold	_____ Reps _____ Sets _____ X Day _____ Hold

65 Notes:

66 Notes:

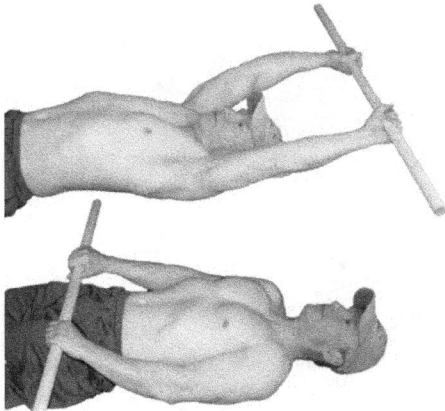

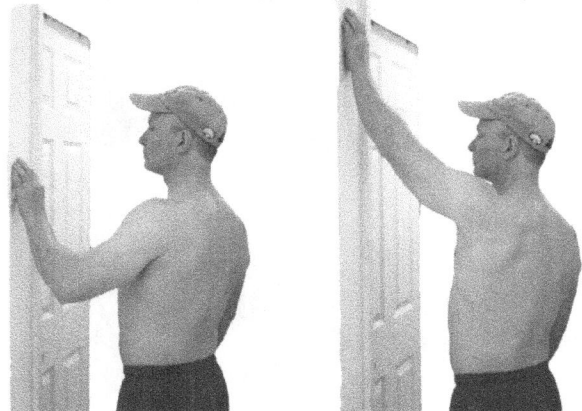

FLEXION - SUPINE - DOWEL

Lie on your back and hold a dowel/cane. Slowly raise the dowel overhead.

*If you have a weak or injured arm, you can use your unaffected arm to assist with the movement.

WALL WALK

Place your target hand on the wall with the palm facing the wall. Walk your fingers up the wall towards overhead. Slide or walk your hand back down the wall to the starting position.

_____ Reps _____ Sets _____ X Day _____ Hold	_____ Reps _____ Sets _____ X Day _____ Hold

67 Notes:

68 Notes:

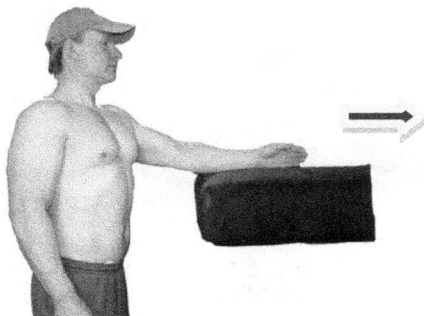

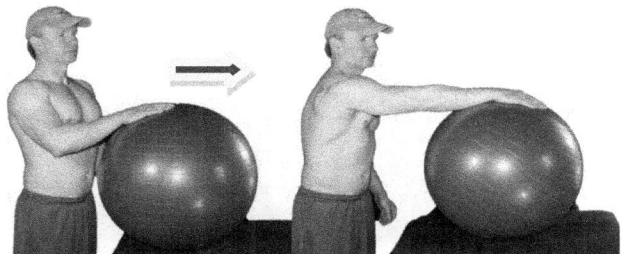

FLEXION - TABLE SLIDE

Sit or stand and rest your target arm on a table and gently slide it forward and then back.

FLEXION - TABLE SLIDE - BALL

Stand and rest your target arm on top of a ball on a table. Gently roll the ball forward and then back.

Shoulder External Rotation (ER)

	_____ Reps _____ Sets _____ X Day _____ Hold		_____ Reps _____ Sets _____ X Day _____ Hold
69	**Notes:**	**70**	**Notes:**

Starting
Position

EXTERNAL ROTATION - SUPINE – DOWEL
INTERNAL ROTATION ON OPPOSITE ARM

Lie on your back holding a dowel/cane with both hands. On the target side, maintain approx. 90-degree bend at the elbow with your arm approximately 30-45 degrees away from your side. Use your other arm to push the dowel/cane to rotate the affected arm back into a stretch. Hold and then return to starting position. Repeat

EXTERNAL ROTATION - 90-90 - DOWEL

Lie on your back and hold a dowel with your elbows out to the side and rested down. Roll your arms back towards overhead until a stretch is felt. Keep elbows bent at a 90-degree angle.

	_____ Reps _____ Sets _____ X Day _____ Hold		_____ Reps _____ Sets _____ X Day _____ Hold
71	**Notes:**	**72**	**Notes:**

EXTERNAL ROTATION – SEATED – DOWEL
INTERNAL ROTATION ON OPPOSITE ARM

Using the unaffected arm, push the dowel into the hand of the target arm. Keep the arm at a 90-degree angle and push until a stretch is felt. Hold and repeat.

EXTERNAL ROTATION – STANDING – DOWEL
INTERNAL ROTATION ON OPPOSITE ARM

Using the unaffected arm, push the dowel into the hand of the target arm. Keep the arm at a 90-degree angle and push until a stretch is felt. Hold and repeat.

Shoulder Internal Rotation (IR) - *also see #69, 71, 72*

	_____ Reps _____ Sets _____X Day _____Hold		_____ Reps _____ Sets _____X Day _____Hold
73	Notes:	**74**	Notes:

INTERNAL ROTATION – TOWEL OR STRAP

Hold one end of the towel in front and with the target arm behind your back. Gently pull up your target arm behind your back with the assist of a towel.

INTERNAL ROTATION – DOWEL

Hold a dowel/cane behind your back. Slowly pull the target arm towards the center of your back.

Shoulder Abduction

	_____ Reps _____ Sets _____X Day _____Hold		_____ Reps _____ Sets _____X Day _____Hold
75	Notes:	**76**	Notes:

ABDUCTION - TABLE SLIDE - BALL

Stand and rest your target arm on top of a ball on a table and gently roll it to the side and back.

ABDUCTION WITH DOWEL

Hold a dowel/cane in front. Slowly push the dowel of the unaffected arm towards the target arm upward and to the side.

Shoulder Extension

	_____ Reps _____ Sets _____X Day _____Hold		_____ Reps _____ Sets _____X Day _____Hold
77	Notes:	**78**	Notes:

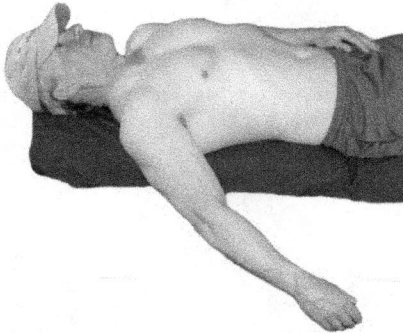

LYING DOWN EXTENSION - TABLE or BED

Lie on your back and gently let target arm drop off table or bed.

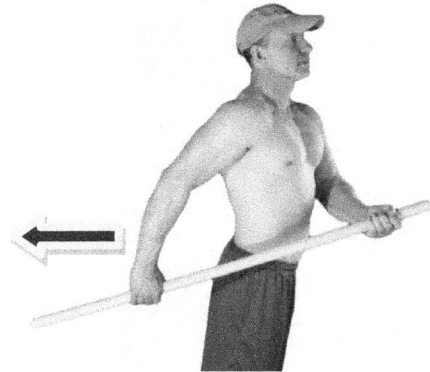

WAND EXTENSION - STANDING

Stand and hold a dowel/cane. Use the unaffected arm to help push the target arm back. The elbow should remain straight the entire time.

Chest/Pec Stretch

	_____ Reps _____ Sets _____X Day _____Hold		_____ Reps _____ Sets _____X Day _____Hold
79	Notes:	**80**	Notes:

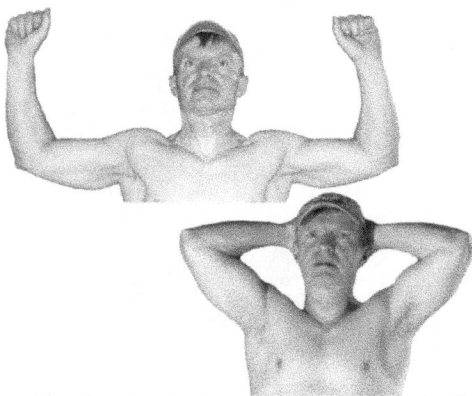

CHEST STRETCH – SEATED, STANDING, or SUPINE

TOP: Bend arms at a 90-degree angle. Move elbows back until feeling a stretch in front of shoulders/chest.

BOTTOM: Clasp hands in back of head. Move elbows back until feeling a stretch in front of shoulders/chest.

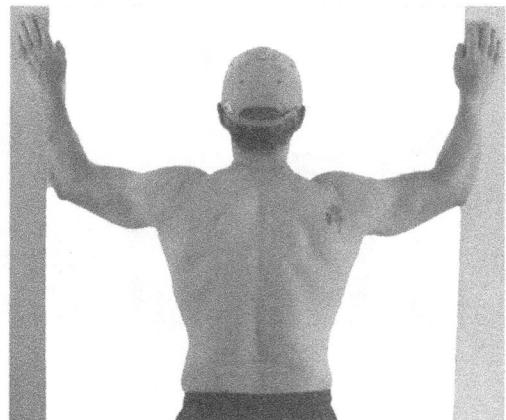

CHEST STRETCH - STEP THROUGH

Stand with arms in doorway at a 90-degree angle. Step through until you feel a stretch through the chest and hold. Keep shoulders down and back. Take another step to increase stretch.

Triceps

	_____ Reps _____ Sets _____X Day _____Hold		_____ Reps _____ Sets _____X Day _____Hold
81	Notes:	**82**	Notes:

TRICEP STRETCH

With your target elbow bent and shoulder raised, use your other hand and gently push your target elbow back towards overhead until a stretch is felt.

TRICEP STRETCH - STRAP or TOWEL

Hold strap of target arm with your hand above your head. Use the other hand to pull downward on the strap, allowing the elbow to bend until a stretch is in the back of the arm.

Posterior Capsule

	_____ Reps _____ Sets _____X Day _____Hold		_____ Reps _____ Sets _____X Day _____Hold
83	Notes:	**84**	Notes:

POSTERIOR SHOULDER/DELTOID RELEASE

Bring your target arm across your body. Use the opposite hand to grasp the back of your shoulder and further pull the arm. Hold.

POSTERIOR CAPSULE STRETCH

Lie on your side and grasp the elbow of the arm closest to the floor. Gently pull it upward and across the front of your body.

Core / Stability Training

Core strengthening is the foundation of all the other exercises that follow, especially balance. Core training is not only an important step in conditioning, but also helps other issues, including neurological, orthopedic, weight, or overall weakness

The core includes muscles of the thoraco-lumbar spine (trunk), cervical spine., erector spinae, abdomen, pelvis, shoulder/scapulae, and your lower lats.

Static core functionality is the ability of one's core to align the skeleton to resist a force that does not change. The core is used to stabilize the thorax and the pelvis during dynamic movement. The nature of dynamic movement must consider our skeletal structure (as a lever) in addition to the force of external resistance and consequently incorporates a vastly different complex of muscles and joints versus a static position.

The core is traditionally assumed to originate most full-body functional movement, including most sports. In addition, the core determines to a large part a person's posture. In all, human anatomy is built to take force upon the bones and direct autonomic force, through various joints, in the desired direction. The core muscles align the spine, ribs, and pelvis of a person to resist a specific force, whether static or dynamic. (Wikipedia: *https://en.wikipedia.org/wiki/Core_(anatomy)*)

These muscles work as stabilizers for the entire body. Core training is simply doing specific exercises to develop and strengthen these stabilizer muscles. If any of these core muscles are weakened, it could result in lower back pain or a protruding waistline. Keeping these core muscles strong can do wonders for your posture and help give you more strength in other exercises like running and walking. (Bodybuilding.com - *https://www.bodybuilding.com/fun/mielke12.htm*)

There is a saying 'form follows function'. This is especially true with core stability and how it affects your balance. Gravity influences all movement, so effective core training must be done against gravity. The rectus abdominus muscle that you are isolating with those crunches flexes the spine/abs only when you are lying on your back or returning the torso to an upright position from hyperextension in standing. "In the upright position, flexion is controlled by eccentric contraction of the back extensors as the lower the weight of the torso in the same direction as gravity". (*Bryant & Green, 2003, p. 84*)

Being able to engage the core with not only your balance exercises but also arm and leg exercises will help prevent injury.

Step 1: First learn to brace the abdomen *(see pictures 1 and 2 on next page)* Think of this as trying to either brace for a punch to the stomach or trying to put on a tight pair of pants (not just sucking in your stomach)

Step 2: After getting a good feel for bracing, try doing a pelvic tilt *(see pictures 3 and 4 on next page)* and then progress to bridging *(see picture 5)*

Step 3: These two basic movements should be done while you progress your abdominal and core training, continuing through the balance section, and to some extent with arm and leg strengthening.

*** When doing floor work, such as crunches, make sure you are on a soft surface, such as a mat, Bosu, stability ball, etc. Pushing your back into a hard surface, such as a wood floor, can do more damage than good to the spine.

*** Breathe – Never hold your breath.

EXERCISE	EXERCISE NUMBER	NOTES
Core / Stability		
ABDOMINAL BRACING TRAINING	1	
ABDOMINAL BRACING - SUPINE	2	
PELVIC TILT - SUPINE	3	
PELVIC TILT - KNEELING	4	
BRIDGING	5	
BRIDGE - BOSU	6	
BRIDGING WITH PILLOW SQUEEZE	7	
BRIDGING WITH PILLOW SQUEEZE - BOSU	8	
BRACE SUPINE MARCHING / BRIDGE LEG UP	9	
BRIDGE LEG UP - BOSU -	10	
SINGLE LEG BRIDGE	11	
BRIDGE SINGLE LEG - BOSU	12	
BRIDGING CROSSED LEG	13	
BRIDGING CROSSED LEG – BOSU	14	
BRIDGING CROSSED LEG - ARMS UP	15	
BRIDGING CROSSED LEG - ARMS UP - BOSU	16	
BRIDGE - ELASTIC BAND	17	
BRIDGING - ABDUCTION - ELASTIC BAND	18	
FLOOR BRIDGE - EXERCISE BALL	19	
FLOOR BRIDGE ALTERNATE LEG LIFT - EXERCISE BALL	20	
BRIDGE UPPER BACK - EXERCISE BALL	21	
BRIDGE UPPER BACK - SINGLE LEG - EXERCISE BALL	22	
QUADRUPED ALTERNATE ARM	23	
QUADRUPED ALTERNATE LEG	24	
QUADRUPED ALTERNATE ARM AND LEG	25	
BIRD DOG ELBOW TOUCHES	26	

EXERCISE Core / Stability	EXERCISE NUMBER	NOTES
PRONE BALL	27	
PRONE BALL - ALTERNATE ARM	28	
PRONE BALL - ALTERNATE LEG	29	
PRONE BALL - ALTERNATE ARM AND LEG	30	
MODIFIED PLANK	31	
MODIFIED PLANK - ALTERNATE LEG	32	
FULL PLANK	33	
PLANK - ALTERNATE ARMS	34	
PLANK - ALTERNATE LEGS	35	
PLANK - EXERCISE BALL	36	
PRONE ON ELBOWS	37	
PRESS UPS	38	
SKYDIVER	39	
PRONE SUPERMAN - BOSU	40	
TRUNK EXTENSION - BOSU	41	
TRUNK EXTENSION - HANDS CROSSED IN FRONT - BOSU	43	
SUPERMAN - ARMS BACK- EXERCISE BALL	44	
SUPERMAN – BOTH ARMS IN FRONT - EXERCISE BALL	45	
SUPERMAN – ONE ARM FORWARD / ONE ARM BACK - EXERCISE BALL	46	
LATERAL PLANK MODIFIED	47	
LATERAL PLANK MODIFIED- BOSU	48	
LATERAL PLANK - 1 KNEE 1 FOOT	49	
LATERAL PLANK - 1 KNEE 1 FOOT – BOSU	50	
LATERAL PLANK	51	
LATERAL PLANK - BOSU	52	

EXERCISE	EXERCISE NUMBER	NOTES
Core / Stability		
LEAN BACK	53	
LEAN BACK - BOSU	54	
LEAN BACK WITH ARMS OUT	55	
LEAN BACK WITH ARMS OUT - BOSU	56	
LEAN BACK WITH TWIST	57	
LEAN BACK WITH TWIST – BOSU	58	
CRUNCHY FROG	59	
SEATED BIKE - FORWARD AND BACKWARDS	60	
CRUNCH – ARMS OUT	61	
CRUNCH – ARMS OUT - BOSU	62	
CRUNCH – ARMS IN BACK OF HEAD	63	
CRUNCH – ARMS IN BACK OF HEAD - BOSU	64	
OBLIQUE CRUNCH	65	
OBLIQUE CRUNCH - BOSU	66	
90 DEGREE CRUNCH	67	
BALL CRUNCH – Can put legs on seat of chair	68	
CURL UPS – ARMS ON LEGS - EXERCISE BALL	69	
CURL UPS- ARMS CROSSED IN FRONT - EXERCISE BALL	70	
CURL UPS – ARMS BEHIND HEAD - EXERCISE BALL	71	
SUPINE CRUNCH TOUCH - EXERCISE BALL	72	
LOWER ABDOMINAL CRUNCH – WITH or WITHOUT BALL	73	
HIGH MARCH CRUNCH	74	
STANDING SIDE CRUNCH	75	
STANDING BIKE CRUNCH	76	

Core/Abdominal

Abdominal Bracing – Pelvic Tilt

	_____ Reps _____ Sets _____X Day _____Hold		_____ Reps _____ Sets _____X Day _____Hold
1	Notes:	**2**	Notes:

ABDOMINAL BRACING TRAINING

Press your fingertips into your relaxed abdomen lateral of your navel. Tighten and brace your abdomen so that the muscles push your fingertips away from the center of your body. Hold, relax and repeat.
Think of this as trying to either brace for a punch to the stomach or trying to put on a tight pair of pants (not just sucking in your stomach)

Starting Position

ABDOMINAL BRACING - SUPINE

Lie on your back. Tighten your stomach muscles as you draw your navel down towards the floor.

Think of this as trying to either brace for a punch to the stomach or trying to put on a tight pair of pants (not just sucking in your stomach)

	_____ Reps _____ Sets _____X Day _____Hold		_____ Reps _____ Sets _____X Day _____Hold
3	Notes:	**4**	Notes:

Starting Position

PELVIC TILT - SUPINE

Lie on your back with your knees bent. Next, arch your low back and then flatten it repeatedly (bracing as above). Your pelvis should tilt forward and back during the movement. Move through a comfortable range of motion.

Starting Position

PELVIC TILT - KNEELING

Kneel on the floor (you can kneel on a pillow or pad if needed). Arch your lower back and then flatten it repeatedly (bracing as above). Your pelvis should tilt forward and back during the movement. Move through a comfortable range of motion.

Bridging

	_____ Reps _____ Sets ____X Day _____Hold		_____ Reps _____ Sets ____X Day _____Hold
5	**Notes:**	**6**	**Notes:**

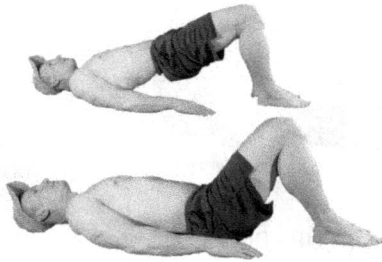

Starting

Position

BRIDGING

Lie on your back. Tighten your lower abdominals (as with abdominal bracing), squeeze your buttocks and then raise your buttocks off the floor/bed. Hold and then lower yourself slowly and repeat. Brace the stomach muscles to keep your spine from moving, trying to keep the pelvis level the entire time.

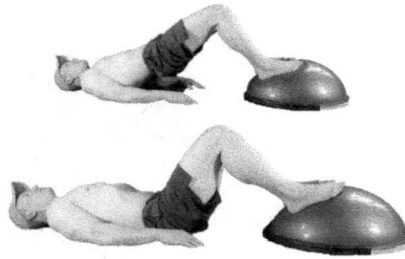

Starting

Position

BRIDGE - BOSU – Can use foam pad, stair step or box

Lie on your back with your feet planted on top of the Bosu and knees bent. Lift up your buttocks as shown. Hold and then lower yourself slowly and repeat.
Brace the stomach muscles to keep your spine from moving, trying to keep the pelvis level the entire time.

	_____ Reps _____ Sets ____X Day _____Hold		_____ Reps _____ Sets ____X Day _____Hold
7	**Notes:**	**8**	**Notes:**

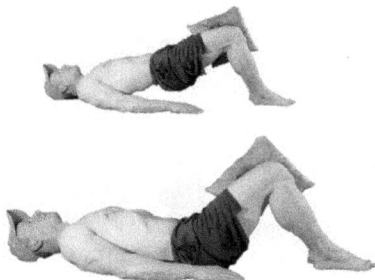

Starting

Position

BRIDGING WITH PILLOW SQUEEZE - Use pillow, ball or rolled towel between knees

Lie on your back and place a pillow, towel roll or ball between your knees and squeeze. Hold this and then tighten your lower abdominals, squeeze your buttocks and raise your buttocks off the floor/bed. Brace the stomach muscles to keep your spine from moving, trying to keep the pelvis level.

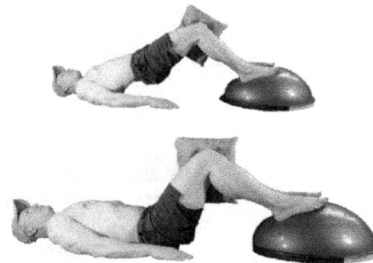

Starting

Position

BRIDGING WITH PILLOW SQUEEZE - BOSU - Can use foam pad, stair step or box

Lie on your back with your feet planted on top of the Bosu and knees bent. Place a pillow, towel roll or ball between your knees and squeeze. Lift up your buttocks as shown. Hold and then lower yourself slowly and repeat. Brace the stomach muscles to keep your spine from moving, trying to keep the pelvis level.

_____ Reps _____ Sets _____ X Day _____ Hold

9	Notes:

Starting
Position

BRACE SUPINE MARCHING / BRIDGE LEG UP

Lie on your back with your knees bent, slowly lift up one foot a few inches and then set it back down. Perform on your other leg. Brace the stomach muscles to keep your spine from moving, trying to keep the pelvis level the entire time.
*To increase challenge, go into bridge position as with #5, then continue march – can bring leg higher to advance

_____ Reps _____ Sets _____ X Day _____ Hold

10	Notes:

Starting
Position

BRIDGE LEG UP - BOSU - Can use foam pad, stair step or box

Lie on your back with your feet planted on top of the Bosu and knees bent. Slowly lift up one foot a few inches and then set it back down. Next, perform on your other leg. Brace the stomach muscles to keep your spine from moving, trying to keep the pelvis level the entire time. *To increase challenge, go into bridge position as with #6, then continue march – can bring leg higher to advance

_____ Reps _____ Sets _____ X Day _____ Hold

11	Notes:

Starting
Position

SINGLE LEG BRIDGE

Lie on your back, raise your buttocks off the floor/bed into a bridge position. Straighten a leg so that only one leg is supporting your body. Then, return that leg back to the ground and change to the other side.   Brace the stomach muscles to keep your spine from moving, trying to keep the pelvis level the entire time.

_____ Reps _____ Sets _____ X Day _____ Hold

12	Notes:

Starting
Position

BRIDGE SINGLE LEG - BOSU - can use foam pad, stair step or box

Lie on your back with your feet planted on top of the Bosu and knees bent, lift up your buttocks and then straighten one knee in the air. Return that leg back to the ground and change to the other side. Brace the stomach muscles to keep your spine from moving, trying to keep the pelvis level the entire time.

	_____ Reps _____ Sets _____ X Day _____ Hold		_____ Reps _____ Sets _____ X Day _____ Hold
13	**Notes:**	**14**	**Notes:**

Starting Position

BRIDGING CROSSED LEG

Lie on your back, cross your leg. Tighten your lower abdomen, squeeze your buttocks and raise your buttocks off the floor/bed. Brace the stomach muscles to keep your spine from moving, trying to keep the pelvis level the entire time.

Starting Position

BRIDGING CROSSED LEG – BOSU - can use foam pad, stair step or box

Lie on your back with your feet planted on top of the Bosu cross your leg. Tighten your lower abdomen, squeeze your buttocks and raise your buttocks. Brace the stomach muscles to keep your spine from moving, trying to keep the pelvis level the entire time.

	_____ Reps _____ Sets _____ X Day _____ Hold		_____ Reps _____ Sets _____ X Day _____ Hold
15	**Notes:**	**16**	**Notes:**

Starting Position

BRIDGING CROSSED LEG - ARMS UP

Lie on your back, cross your leg and put your hands together as shown. Next, tighten your lower abdomen, squeeze your buttocks and raise your buttocks off the floor/bed. Brace the stomach muscles to keep your spine from moving, trying to keep the pelvis level the entire time.

BRIDGING CROSSED LEG - ARMS UP - BOSU - can use foam pad, stair step or box

Lie on your back with your feet planted on top of the Bosu and hands together and leg crossed. Tighten your lower abdomen, squeeze your buttocks and raise your buttocks. Brace the stomach muscles to keep your spine from moving, trying to keep the pelvis level.

	_____ Reps _____ Sets _____ X Day _____ Hold		_____ Reps _____ Sets _____ X Day _____ Hold
17	**Notes:**	**18**	**Notes:**

Starting Position

BRIDGE - ELASTIC BAND

Lie on your back, hold an elastic band down around your waist for resistance. Tighten your lower abdomen, squeeze your buttocks and then raise your buttocks off the floor/bed. Brace the stomach muscles to keep your spine from moving, trying to keep the pelvis level the entire time.

Starting Position

BRIDGING - ABDUCTION - ELASTIC BAND – can be done with feet on BOSU, foam, stair step or box

Lie on your back, place an elastic band around your knees and pull your knees apart. Hold this and then tighten your lower abdomen, squeeze your buttocks and raise your buttocks off the floor/bed. Brace the stomach muscles to keep your spine from moving, trying to keep the pelvis level the entire time.

	_____ Reps _____ Sets _____ X Day _____ Hold		_____ Reps _____ Sets _____ X Day _____ Hold
19	**Notes:**	**20**	**Notes:**

Starting Position

FLOOR BRIDGE - EXERCISE BALL

Lie on the floor, place an exercise ball under your lower legs and then raise up your buttocks. Hold and repeat. Brace the stomach muscles to keep your spine from moving, trying to keep the pelvis level the entire time.

Starting Position

FLOOR BRIDGE ALTERNATE LEG LIFT - EXERCISE BALL

Lie on the floor, place an exercise ball under your lower legs and then raise up your buttocks. While holding this position raise up a leg off the ball towards the ceiling then lower back to the ball and alternate to lift the other leg. Brace the stomach muscles to keep your spine from moving, trying to keep the pelvis level.

		_____ Reps _____ Sets _____ X Day _____ Hold
21	**Notes:**	

BRIDGE UPPER BACK - EXERCISE BALL

Start in a seated position on the ball and slowly walk your feet forward so that the ball is on your upper back. Keep your buttocks and pelvis up off the ball and straight with your thighs. Brace the stomach muscles to keep your spine from moving, trying to keep the pelvis level the entire time.
*To increase the challenge, you can do a supine march or perform some arm exercises, such as Fly's or Chest Presses (_See Upper Extremity exercises_)

		_____ Reps _____ Sets _____ X Day _____ Hold
22	**Notes:**	

Starting Position

BRIDGE UPPER BACK - SINGLE LEG - EXERCISE BALL

Start in a seated position on the ball and slowly walk your feet forward so that the ball is on your upper back. Keep your buttocks and pelvis up off the ball and straight with your thighs. Raise up one leg so that you straighten your knee in the air. Return it back to the floor and then switch to raise up the other side. Brace the stomach muscles to keep your spine from moving, trying to keep the pelvis level the entire time.

Quadruped

		_____ Reps _____ Sets _____ X Day _____ Hold
23	**Notes:**	

QUADRUPED ALTERNATE ARM

While in a crawling position, slowly raise up an arm out in front of you.

		_____ Reps _____ Sets _____ X Day _____ Hold
24	**Notes:**	

QUADRUPED ALTERNATE LEG

While in a crawling position, slowly draw your leg back behind you as you straighten your knee. Either repeat on same side or alternate.

_____ Reps _____ Sets _____X Day _____Hold

25

Notes:

QUADRUPED ALTERNATE ARM AND LEG

While in a crawling position, brace at your abdominals and then slowly lift a leg and opposite arm upwards. Maintain a level and stable pelvis and spine the entire time. Either repeat on same side or alternate.

_____ Reps _____ Sets _____X Day _____Hold

26

Notes:

Touch your elbow to your opposite knee

Starting Position

BIRD DOG ELBOW TOUCHES

While in a crawling position, slowly lift your leg and opposite arm upwards. When returning your arm and leg down, do not touch the floor but instead touch your elbow to your opposite knee and lift and straighten them again. Then set them down on the floor. Either repeat on same side or alternate.

_____ Reps _____ Sets _____X Day _____Hold

27

Notes:

PRONE BALL

Lie face down over a ball, support your self with your feet and hands.

_____ Reps _____ Sets _____X Day _____Hold

28

Notes:

PRONE BALL - ALTERNATE ARM

Lie face down over a ball, support your self with your feet and hands. Next, slowly raise up one arm. Return arm back to floor and then raise up the other arm. Keep alternating arms.

	_____ Reps _____ Sets _____ X Day _____ Hold		_____ Reps _____ Sets _____ X Day _____ Hold
29	Notes:	**30**	Notes:

PRONE BALL - ALTERNATE LEG

Lie face down over a ball, support yourself with your arms and legs. Next slowly raise up a leg. Return leg back to floor and then raise up the other leg.

PRONE BALL - ALTERNATE ARM AND LEG

Lie face down over a ball, support yourself with your feet and hands. Next, slowly raise up one arm and opposite leg. Return arm and leg back to floor and then raise up the opposite arm/leg.

Plank

	_____ Reps _____ Sets _____ X Day _____ Hold		_____ Reps _____ Sets _____ X Day _____ Hold
31	Notes:	**32**	Notes:

MODIFIED PLANK

Lie face down, lift your body up on your elbows and toes. Try and maintain a straight spine the entire time. Do not allow your low back sag downward.

Starting

Position

MODIFIED PLANK - ALTERNATE LEG

Lie face down, lift your body up on your elbows and toes. Next, lift one leg off the ground and then set it back down. Then repeat on the other leg. Try and maintain a straight spine the entire time.

_____ Reps _____ Sets _____ X Day _____ Hold

33 | Notes:

FULL PLANK

Lie face down, lift your body up on your elbows and toes. Straighten your arms in full elbow extension and hold in full plank position. Do not let your back arch down. Try and maintain a straight spine the entire time.

_____ Reps _____ Sets _____ X Day _____ Hold

34 | Notes:

PLANK - ALTERNATE ARMS

Hold a plank position as previous (#33). Raise one arm out in front of you as shown. Return to the starting position and then raise your other arm out in front of you and repeat.
Try and maintain a straight spine the entire time.

_____ Reps _____ Sets _____ X Day _____ Hold

35 | Notes:

PLANK - ALTERNATE LEGS

Hold a plank position as previous (#33). Raise one leg off the floor as shown. Return to the starting position and then raise your other leg and repeat. Try and maintain a straight spine the entire time.

_____ Reps _____ Sets _____ X Day _____ Hold

36 | Notes:

PLANK - EXERCISE BALL

While kneeling on the floor with an exercise ball in front of you, place your elbows and hands on the ball and lift your body up. Try and maintain a straight spine. Do not allow your hips or pelvis on either side to drop.

Back Extension

_____ Reps _____ Sets _____ X Day _____ Hold	_____ Reps _____ Sets _____ X Day _____ Hold
37 Notes:	**38** Notes:

PRONE ON ELBOWS

Lie face down, slowly press up and prop yourself up on your elbows.

PRESS UPS

Lie face down, slowly press up and arch your back using your arms.

_____ Reps _____ Sets _____ X Day _____ Hold	_____ Reps _____ Sets _____ X Day _____ Hold
39 Notes:	**40** Notes:

SKYDIVER

Lie face down with arms by your side. Next, lift your upper body, lower legs, thighs, and arms off the ground at the same time as shown. You can place a pillow under your stomach/hips for comfort.

PRONE SUPERMAN - BOSU

Lie face down over the Bosu. Slowly raise your arms and legs upward off the ground. Then lower slowly back to the ground.

_____ Reps _____ Sets _____ X Day _____ Hold

41

Notes:

TRUNK EXTENSION - BOSU

Lie face down with your upper body on a Bosu and slowly raise your head and chest upwards as shown.
Your arms can be behind your back or alongside your body.

_____ Reps _____ Sets _____ X Day _____ Hold

42

Notes:

TRUNK EXTENSION - HANDS BEHIND HEAD - BOSU

Lie face down with your upper body on a Bosu. Touch the back of your head with both hands and slowly raise your head and chest upwards.

_____ Reps _____ Sets _____ X Day _____ Hold

43

Notes:

TRUNK EXTENSION - HANDS CROSSED IN FRONT - BOSU

While lying face down with your upper body on a Bosu, slowly raise your head and chest upwards.
Keep your arms crossed on your chest as you perform.

_____ Reps _____ Sets _____ X Day _____ Hold

44

Notes:

SUPERMAN - ARMS BACK- EXERCISE BALL

Start in a kneeling position with an exercise ball in front of you. Roll forward so that you are face down on the ball with your feet on the ground and your stomach on the ball. Hold up your head and chest so that a straight line exists between your feet and head. Also bring your arms back along side of your body and hold this position.

_____ Reps _____ Sets _____ X Day _____ Hold		_____ Reps _____ Sets _____ X Day _____ Hold
45	**Notes:**	**46**	**Notes:**

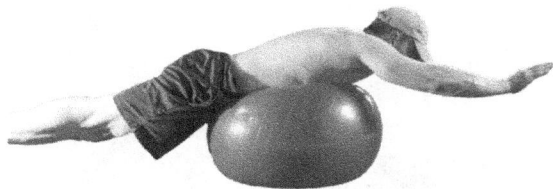

SUPERMAN – BOTH ARMS IN FRONT - EXERCISE BALL

Start in a kneeling position with an exercise ball in front of you. Next, roll forward so that you are face down on the ball with your feet on the ground and your stomach on the ball. Hold up your head and chest so that a straight line exists between your feet and head. Also bring your arms up and forward out in front of you and hold this position.

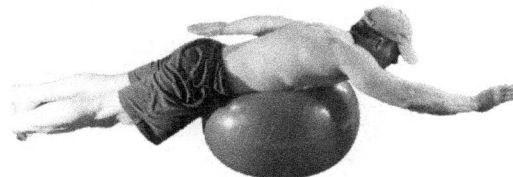

SUPERMAN – ONE ARM FORWARD / ONE ARM BACK - EXERCISE BALL

Start in a kneeling position with an exercise ball in front of you. Next, roll forward so that you are face down on the ball with your feet on the ground and your stomach on the ball. Hold up your head and chest so that a straight line exists between your feet and head. Raise one arm up and out in front of you as you bring the other arm back and along side your body as in a swimming motion.

Lateral Plank

_____ Reps _____ Sets _____ X Day _____ Hold		_____ Reps _____ Sets _____ X Day _____ Hold
47	**Notes:**	**48**	**Notes:**

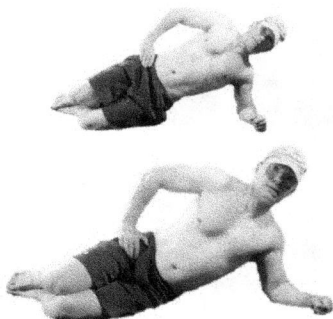

Starting Position

LATERAL PLANK MODIFIED

Lie on your side with your knees bent, lift your body up on your elbow and knees. Try and maintain a straight spine.

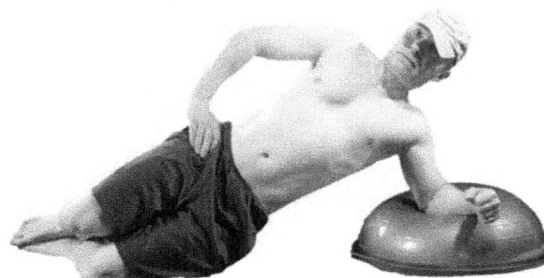

LATERAL PLANK MODIFIED- BOSU- can be anything unstable

Lie on your side with your knees bent and your elbow on the Bosu, lift your body up on your elbow and knees. Try and maintain a straight spine.

	_____ Reps _____ Sets _____X Day _____Hold
49	**Notes:**

LATERAL PLANK - 1 KNEE 1 FOOT

Lie on your side with bottom knee bent and top knee straight. Lift your body up on your elbow and knee on one side and foot on the other side. Try and maintain a straight spine.

	_____ Reps _____ Sets _____X Day _____Hold
50	**Notes:**

LATERAL PLANK - 1 KNEE 1 FOOT – BOSU- Can be anything unstable

Lie on your side with elbow on Bosu with bottom knee bent and the top knee straight. Lift your body up on your elbow and knee on one side and foot on the other side. Try and maintain a straight spine.

	_____ Reps _____ Sets _____X Day _____Hold
51	**Notes:**

Starting

Position

LATERAL PLANK

Lie on your side with both legs straight and lift your body up on your elbow and feet. Try and maintain a straight spine.

	_____ Reps _____ Sets _____X Day _____Hold
52	**Notes:**

LATERAL PLANK - BOSU - Can be anything unstable

Lie on your side with your elbow on the Bosu and both legs straight. Lift your body up on your elbow and feet. Try and maintain a straight spine.

Backward Lean

_____ Reps _____ Sets _____X Day _____Hold	_____ Reps _____ Sets _____X Day _____Hold
53 Notes:	**54** Notes:

LEAN BACK

Start in an upright seated position with knees bent. Hold onto thighs and lean back keeping spine as straight as possible.

LEAN BACK - BOSU

Start in an upright seated position on Bosu with knees bent. Hold onto thighs or Bosu and lean back keeping spine as straight as possible.

_____ Reps _____ Sets _____X Day _____Hold	_____ Reps _____ Sets _____X Day _____Hold
55 Notes:	**56** Notes:

LEAN BACK WITH ARMS OUT

Start in an upright seated position with knees bent. Hold arms straight out or overhead, brace core and lean back keeping spine as straight as possible

LEAN BACK WITH ARMS OUT - BOSU

Start in an upright seated position on Bosu with knees bent. Hold arms straight out or overhead, brace core and lean back keeping spine as straight as possible.

	_____ Reps _____ Sets _____ X Day _____ Hold		_____ Reps _____ Sets _____ X Day _____ Hold
57	**Notes:**	**58**	**Notes:**

Starting

Position

LEAN BACK WITH TWIST

Start in an upright seated position with knees bent. Hold arms straight out, brace core and lean back keeping spine as straight as possible. Rotate trunk/arms to one side and then repeat to the other side.

Starting

Position

LEAN BACK WITH TWIST – BOSU

Start in an upright seated position on Bosu with knees bent. Hold arms straight out, brace core and lean back keeping spine as straight as possible. Rotate trunk/arms to one side - repeat to the other side

	_____ Reps _____ Sets _____ X Day _____ Hold		_____ Reps _____ Sets _____ X Day _____ Hold
59	**Notes:**	**60**	**Notes:**

CRUNCHY FROG

Sit on floor or edge of couch/bench. Lean back and with arms wide apart and legs straight. Next, bring knees towards chest and arms forward and return to starting position.

SEATED BIKE - FORWARD AND BACKWARDS

Sit on floor and lean back. With arms on floor or off ground, peddle feet forward for 15-30 repetitions, rest and then reverse. *Progress by moving hands forward near hips or remove arm support*

Abdominal Crunch Variations

_____ Reps _____ Sets _____ X Day _____ Hold

61 | Notes:

Starting
Position

CRUNCH – ARMS OUT

Lie on your back with your arms outstretched forward, brace core and curl up lifting your shoulder blades off the ground. Exhale as you come up and squeeze/tighten your abdominal muscles.

_____ Reps _____ Sets _____ X Day _____ Hold

62 | Notes:

Starting
Position

CRUNCH – ARMS OUT - BOSU

Lie on your back on Bosu with your arms outstretched forward, brace core and curl up lifting your shoulder blades off the ground. Exhale as you come up and squeeze/tighten your abdominal muscles.

_____ Reps _____ Sets _____ X Day _____ Hold

63 | Notes:

Starting
Position

CRUNCH – ARMS IN BACK OF HEAD

Lie on your back with your arms behind your head, brace core and curl up lifting your shoulder blades off the ground. Exhale as you come up and squeeze/tighten your abdominal muscles. Do not pull on your neck/head.

_____ Reps _____ Sets _____ X Day _____ Hold

64 | Notes:

CRUNCH – ARMS IN BACK OF HEAD - BOSU

Lie on your back on Bosu with your arms behind your head, brace core and curl up lifting your shoulder blades off the ground. Exhale as you come up and squeeze/tighten your abdominal muscles. Do not pull on your neck/head.

	_____ Reps _____ Sets _____X Day _____Hold
65	**Notes:**

OBLIQUE CRUNCH

Lie on your back with one or both hands in back of head. Brace core and curl up targeting elbow to opposite knee as shown. Keep shoulders off floor. Exhale as you come up and squeeze/tighten your abdominal muscles. Do not pull on your neck/head.

	_____ Reps _____ Sets _____X Day _____Hold
66	**Notes:**

OBLIQUE CRUNCH - BOSU

Lie back on Bosu with one or both hands in back of head. Brace core and curl up targeting elbow to opposite knee as shown. Keep shoulders off Bosu. Exhale as you come up and squeeze/tighten your abdominal muscles. Do not pull on your neck/head.

	_____ Reps _____ Sets _____X Day _____Hold
67	**Notes:**

90 DEGREE CRUNCH

Lie on your back with legs straight in air. Reach your hands towards toes, crunching shoulders off ground. Exhale as you come up and squeeze/tighten your abdominal muscles.

	_____ Reps _____ Sets _____X Day _____Hold
68	**Notes:**

BALL CRUNCH – Can put legs on seat of chair

Lie on back with legs up on ball so knees and hips are at ~ 90 degrees. Cross hands over chest or behind head. Brace core and curl up lifting your shoulder blades off the ground. Exhale as you come up and squeeze/tighten your abdominal muscles. Do not pull on your neck/head.

	_____ Reps _____ Sets _____ X Day _____ Hold
69	**Notes:**

Starting

Position

CURL UPS – ARMS ON LEGS - EXERCISE BALL

While sitting on an exercise ball, roll forward so that your back lies against the ball. Put hands on thighs/legs. Brace core and curl up lifting your shoulder blades off the ball. Exhale as you come up and squeeze/tighten your abdominal muscles.

	_____ Reps _____ Sets _____ X Day _____ Hold
70	**Notes:**

CURL UPS- ARMS CROSSED IN FRONT - EXERCISE BALL

While sitting on an exercise ball, roll forward so that your back lies against the ball. Cross hands over your chest. Brace core and curl up lifting your shoulder blades off the ball. Exhale as you come up and squeeze/tighten your abdominal muscles.

	_____ Reps _____ Sets _____ X Day _____ Hold
71	**Notes:**

CURL UPS – ARMS BEHIND HEAD - EXERCISE BALL

While sitting on an exercise ball, roll forward so that your back lies against the ball. Place your hands behind your head. Brace core and curl up lifting your shoulder blades off the ball. Exhale as you come up and squeeze/tighten your abdominal muscles. Do not pull on your neck/head.

	_____ Reps _____ Sets _____ X Day _____ Hold
72	**Notes:**

Starting   Position

SUPINE CRUNCH TOUCH - EXERCISE BALL

Lie on the floor with your knees bend and holding a ball over your head. Bring both your knees and ball towards each other above your chest and touch your knees to the ball. Slowly return both to original positions and repeat.

_____ Reps _____ Sets _____ X Day _____ Hold

73	Notes:

LOWER ABDOMINAL CRUNCH – WITH or WITHOUT BALL

Sit on a solid surface with or without a ball/pillow between your knees. Maintaining a straight spine, contract your lower abdominals. Lift both knees up. Hold and control movement back to starting position. Repeat. Can be done holding onto surface for added stability with or without ball (3rd picture)

_____ Reps _____ Sets _____ X Day _____ Hold

74	Notes:

HIGH MARCH CRUNCH

Lift knee towards chest keeping hips forward in a high march position. Continue to alternate sides while standing in place. Exhale as you come up and squeeze/tighten your abdominal muscles.

_____ Reps _____ Sets _____ X Day _____ Hold

75	Notes:

Starting Position

STANDING SIDE CRUNCH

Standing with hip rotated out bring knee up towards same side elbow squeezing your obliques. Continue alternating sides while standing in place. Exhale as you come up and squeeze/tighten muscles.

_____ Reps _____ Sets _____ X Day _____ Hold

76	Notes:

Starting Position

STANDING BIKE CRUNCH

Lift knee to chest and rotate pulling opposite elbow towards knee. Continue to alternate sides while standing in place. Exhale as you come up and squeeze/tighten muscles.

Strengthening

Anaerobic - without oxygen: Single repetition with maximum resistance
Lifting lighter weights with a high number of repetitions will result in 'toning', whereas lifting heavier weights with a lower number of repetitions will result in 'bulking up'.

Benefits of strengthening	• Increases muscle fiber size and contractile strength • Increases tendon and ligament strength • Increases bone strength / bone mineral density • Improves hormonal balances-decreased cortisol • Increases Peripheral (PNS) and Central (CNS) Nervous System communication/proprioception • Improves function for ADL's (Activities of Daily Living)
Range of Motion (ROM)	Refers to the distance and direction a joint can move between the flexed position and the extended position (stretching from flexion to extension for physiological gain). It is important to be able to complete full ROM before adding resistance. *Before strengthening (adding resistance), make sure you can go through full ROM* unless being followed by an MD or physical/occupational therapist or other professional.
Forms of strengthening exercise	• **Isometric** – Muscles contract with no motion at the joint or change in length of the muscle. The exercises usually consist of maximal effort against an object that does not move, like a wall. • **Isotonic** – Muscles contract with motion at the joint; muscles either lengthen or shorten (*see concentric/eccentric below*). Tension is not constant through the range of motion. (During a bicep curl, holding a 5 lb weight, the contraction is not constant during the entire movement). Most common form of isotonic exercises use free weights with either dumbbells or a barbell. • **Concentric** – Muscle shortens, positive phase of lift. Bending the elbow in a bicep curl • **Eccentric** – Muscle lengthens, negative phase of lift or lowering. Straightening the elbow in a bicep curl. • **Isokinetic** – Muscles contract with motion at the joint; muscles either lengthen or shorten. Machines or equipment control the speed of the movement, so tension is constant providing the maximum amount of resistance throughout the entire movement.
Repetition (Reps)	Single cycle of lifting and lowering a weight in a controlled manner, moving through the form of the exercise. Example: 12 Bicep curls per set.
Set	Several repetitions performed one after another with no break between. There can be a number of reps per set and sets per exercise depending on the goal of the individual. Example: 12 reps x3 sets
Rep Maximum (RM)	The number of repetitions one can perform at a certain weight is called the Rep Maximum (RM). For example, if one could perform 10 repetitions with a 75 lbs dumbbell, then their RM for that weight would be 10RM. 1RM is the maximum weight that someone can lift in a given exercise - i.e. a weight that they can only lift once. (*Wikipedia*) (*See Bulk Up or Tone Up Below*)
Bulk up or Tone up	Do you want to 'bulk up' or 'tone up'? Although much of this depends on genetics and your ratio of slow and fast twitch fibers, discussed in the *Endurance* section, it is good to know what your goals are before starting. The average person should be able to perform at about 75% of their maximum resistance for 10 repetitions. If you can do ONE bicep curl with a 20-pound dumbbell/weight, then you should be able to do 10 with a 15 lbs. weight. (See *Set*) 20 lbs. x 75% = 15 lbs. Once you get into a routine, it will be easy for you to know when to increase the weight.

General rule of thumb	• Work from the Ground up • Order: Isometric > ROM > Eccentric > Concentric • Use assistance before resistance – Start without weight to complete range of motion and then add weight with proper form. *(See ROM above)* • Add weight: 8-12 reps x 2-3 sets of each exercise at 75% of one repetition maximum (one-rep max). • Once you reach 12 easily, you can then recheck your one-rep max. If it has increased, then increase your weight as above. • If you are looking to 'bulk up', perform low repetitions at a higher weight – up to 85-90% of the one-rep maximum. 5-8 reps x 2-3 sets. With increased weight, there is a higher risk of injury. • If you are looking to 'tone up', perform high repetitions with 65-75% of the one-rep max. 12-20 reps x 2-3 sets. • Do NOT exercise the same muscle group every day. The muscles need about 48-72 hours to repair. This includes the abdomen. **Muscle strengthening, if you are lifting weights, alternate upper and lower body with isolated abdomen exercises every other day as well. For those working out several days a week, find a schedule that works for you, but give each muscle group 48-72 hours to recover. • Cardiac/aerobic conditioning can be done daily. • Breathe!! Always exhale on the exertion. For example, when you are doing a crunch, exhale as you flexing the abs or 'curling'. Do not hold your breath. • Engage your core. Don't forget what you learned under core and balance.

Duration, Frequency, Intensity and Movement Patterns

Intensity: How *much* mental and physical *effort* it takes to sustain an activity.	This can be done using the target heart rate range THR (optimum exercise intensity levels through beats per minute, talk test or rate of perceived exertion.
Duration: How *long* the training lasts.	The higher the intensity, the shorter the duration. The American College of Sports Medicine guidelines recommend all healthy adults aged 18–65 yr should participate in moderate intensity aerobic physical activity for a minimum of 30 min on five days per week, or vigorous intensity aerobic activity for a minimum of 20 min on three days per week.
Frequency: How *often* the training occurs.	Strength training should be performed every other day or 2-3 days a week. It is important to give each muscle group 48-72 hours to recover. Alternate upper and lower body with isolated abdomen/core exercises every other day. For those working out several days a week, find a schedule that works for you as long as you give each muscle group 48 hours of recovery time.

Movement Patterns and Examples
 	
Basic movements that help to increase overall body strengthening
	• Bend and Lift: Squats, Dead Lifts and Leg presses
	   ○ Picking up item off floor
	• Single Leg: Step ups, Single leg stance, Lunges
	   ○ Walking up steps
	• Push: Shoulder press, Bench press, Push up
	   ○ Pushing Shopping cart or Lawn mower
	• Pull: Lat pull downs, Seated rows
	   ○ Vacuuming, Raking
	• Rotational
	   ○ Shoveling snow

EXERCISE Lower Extremity - Lying & Seated Strengthening and Range of Motion	EXERCISE NUMBER	NOTES
INVERSION – SEATED - ELASTIC BAND	1	
INVERSION – SEATED - ELASTIC BAND - 2	2	
EVERSION – SEATED - ELASTIC BAND	3	
EVERSION – SEATED - ELASTIC BAND - 2	4	
ANKLE PUMPS - SEATED	5	
ANKLE PUMPS – SUPINE or FEET UP ON STOOL	6	
DORSIFLEXION – SEATED - ELASTIC BAND	7	
DORSIFLEXION – SEATED - ELASTIC BAND - 2	8	
PLANTARFLEXION - STRAP	9	
PLANTARFLEXION - SEATED – ELASTIC BAND	10	
HEEL SLIDES - SUPINE	11	
HEEL SLIDES - RESISTED EXTENSION – ELASTIC BAND	12	
QUAD SET –ISOMETRIC	13	
QUAD SET WITH TOWEL UNDER HEEL - ISOMETRIC	14	
SHORT ARC QUAD (SAQ) – SELF ASSISTED	15	
SHORT ARC QUAD - (SAQ)	16	
KNEE EXTENSION - SELF ASSISTED	17	
PARTIAL ARC QUAD - LOW SEAT	18	
LONG ARC QUAD (LAQ) – LOW SEAT (90 deg)	19	
LONG ARC QUAD (LAQ) – LOW SEAT - ANKLE WEIGHTS	20	
LONG ARC QUAD (LAQ) - HIGH SEAT	21	
LONG ARC QUAD (LAQ) - HIGH SEAT - ANKLE WEIGHTS	22	
LONG ARC QUAD - ELASTIC BAND – HAND HELD	23	
LONG ARC QUAD - ELASTIC BAND	24	

EXERCISE Lower Extremity - Lying & Seated Strengthening and Range of Motion	EXERCISE NUMBER	NOTES
HAMSTRING CURLS - PRONE - ASSISTED	25	
HAMSTRING CURLS - PRONE	26	
HAMSTRING CURLS - - PRONE - WEIGHTS	27	
HAMSTRING CURLS – PRONE - ELASTIC BAND	28	
HAMSTRING CURLS – ELASTIC BAND	29	
HAMSTRING CURLS – ELASTIC BAND - 2	30	
HAMSTRING CURLS ON BALL	31	
HAMSTRING CURLS - SINGLE LEG - EXERCISE BALL	32	
HIP FLEXION ISOMETRIC	33	
HIP FLEXION ISOMETRIC BILATERAL	34	
HIP FLEXION – ISOMETRIC	35	
STRAIGHT LEG RAISE (SLR)	36	
STRAIGHT LEG RAISE (SLR) – ANKLE WEIGHTS	37	
STRAIGHT LEG RAISE (SLR) - ELASTIC BAND	38	
SEATED MARCHING	39	
SEATED MARCHING - ELASTIC BAND	40	
HIP EXTENSION - PRONE	41	
HIP EXTENSION – PRONE – ANKLE WEIGHTS	42	
HIP EXTENSION – PRONE – ELASTIC BAND	43	
HIP EXTENSION – QUADRUPED	44	
HIP ABDUCTION - SUPINE	45	
HIP ABDUCTION - SUPINE – ANKLE WEIGHTS	46	
HIP ABDUCTION – SUPINE - ELASTIC BAND	47	
HIP ABDUCTION / CLAMS– SUPINE - ELASTIC BAND	48	
MODIFIED HIP ABDUCTION – SIDELYING	49	

EXERCISE Lower Extremity - Lying & Seated Strengthening and Range of Motion	EXERCISE NUMBER	NOTES
HIP ABDUCTION – SIDELYING	50	
HIP ABDUCTION – SIDELYING - WEIGHTS	51	
HIP ABDUCTION – SIDELYING - ELASTIC BAND	52	
CLAM SHELLS	53	
SIDELYING CLAM - ELASTIC BAND	54	
HIP ABDUCTION - FIRE HYDRANT - QUADRUPED	55	
HIP ABDUCTION - FIRE HYDRANT – QUADRUPED - ELASTIC BAND	56	
HIP ABDUCTION - SEATED - STRAIGHT LEG	57	
HIP ABDUCTION - SEATED - STRAIGHT LEG – ANKLE WEIGHT	58	
HIP ABDUCTION - SINGLE- SEATED	59	
HIP ABDUCTION - SINGLE- SEATED – ELASTIC BAND	60	
HIP ABDUCTION - BILATERAL- SEATED	61	
HIP ABDUCTION - BILATERAL- SEATED - ELASTIC BAND	62	
HIP ADDUCTION SQUEEZE – SUPINE – KNEES BENT	63	
HIP ADDUCTION SQUEEZE – SUPINE – LEGS STRAIGHT	64	
HIP ADDUCTION - SIDELYING	65	
INTERNAL ROTATION - HEEL SQUEEZE - ISOMETRIC	67	
HIP INTERNAL ROTATION - SUPINE	68	
REVERSE CLAMS - SIDELYING	69	
REVERSE CLAMS - SIDELYING - ELASTIC BAND	70	
HIP INTERNAL ROTATION - SEATED	71	
HIP INTERNAL ROTATION - ELASTIC BAND	72	
HIP EXTERNAL ROTATION - SUPINE	73	

EXERCISE Lower Extremity - Lying & Seated Strengthening and Range of Motion	EXERCISE NUMBER	NOTES
HIP EXTERNAL ROTATION - ELASTIC BAND	74	
HIP ROTATIONS – BILATERAL - SIDELYING	75	
HIP ROTATION - SEATED - BALL and ELASTIC BAND	76	
PRESS – BILATERAL – ELASTIC BAND	77	
PRESS – SINGLE LEG – ELASTIC BAND	78	
HIP HIKE - STANDING	79	
HIP HIKE – KNEELING	80	
GLUTE SETS - PRONE	81	
GLUTE SET - SUPINE	82	
GLUTE SQUEEZE - SITTING	83	
PT (MAX/MEDIUS)	84	

LOWER EXTREMITY - Range Of Motion > Isometric > Strength
Lying and Seated

Inversion (IV) / Eversion (EV)

1	_____ Reps _____ Sets _____ X Day _____ Hold
	Notes:

2	_____ Reps _____ Sets _____ X Day _____ Hold
	Notes:

INVERSION – SEATED - ELASTIC BAND

In a seated position, cross your legs and using an elastic band attached to your foot, hook it under your opposite foot and up to your hand.   Draw the resisted foot inward. Keep your heel in contact with the floor the entire time.

INVERSION – SEATED - ELASTIC BAND - 2

In a seated position, use an elastic band secured to a steady object and the other end attached to your foot. Draw the resisted foot inward. Keep your heel in contact with the floor the entire time.

3	_____ Reps _____ Sets _____ X Day _____ Hold
	Notes:

4	_____ Reps _____ Sets _____ X Day _____ Hold
	Notes:

EVERSION – SEATED - ELASTIC BAND

In a seated position, use an elastic band attached to your foot, hook it under your opposite foot and up to your hand. Draw the resisted foot outward. Keep your heel in contact with the floor the entire time.

EVERSION – SEATED - ELASTIC BAND - 2

In a seated position, use an elastic band secured to a steady object and the other end attached to your foot. Draw the resisted foot outward. Keep your heel in contact with the floor the entire time.

Dorsiflexion (DF) / Plantarflexion (PF)

_____ Reps _____ Sets _____ X Day _____ Hold	_____ Reps _____ Sets _____ X Day _____ Hold
5 **Notes:**	**6** **Notes:**

ANKLE PUMPS - SEATED

In a seated position keeping feet on the floor, first go up on toes (toes pointed towards the ground – PF). Then point toes up keeping heels on the ground (DF). Alternate back and forth in a pumping motion.

ANKLE PUMPS – SUPINE or FEET UP ON STOOL

Lying or with feet up on stool first point the toes forward (PF) and then back up with toes facing the ceiling. Alternate back and forth in a pumping motion.

_____ Reps _____ Sets _____ X Day _____ Hold	_____ Reps _____ Sets _____ X Day _____ Hold
7 **Notes:**	**8** **Notes:**

DORSIFLEXION – SEATED - ELASTIC BAND

In a seated position, use an elastic band attached to your target foot, hook it under your opposite foot and up to your hand. Draw the band upwards with the resisted foot as shown. Keep your heel in contact with the floor the entire time.

DORSIFLEXION – SEATED - ELASTIC BAND - 2

In a seated position, use an elastic band secured to a steady object and the other end attached to your foot. Draw the resisted foot upward. Keep your heel in contact with the floor the entire time.

_____ Reps	_____ Sets	_____X Day	_____ Hold

9 Notes:

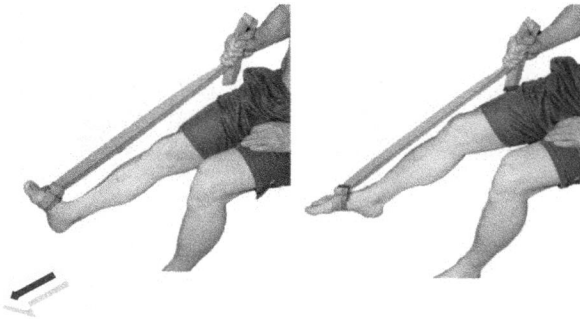

PLANTARFLEXION - STRAP

In a seated position, attach one loop of the strap to your foot and hold the other end. Move your foot forward and back at the ankle as shown. Keep your heel in contact with the floor the entire time.

_____ Reps	_____ Sets	_____X Day	_____ Hold

10 Notes:

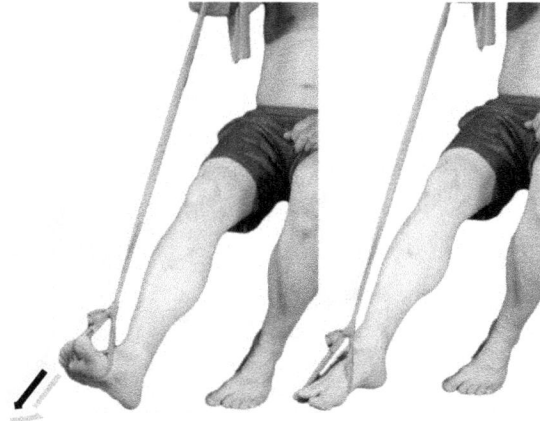

PLANTARFLEXION - SEATED – ELASTIC BAND

In a seated position, hold an elastic band and attach the other end to your foot. Press your foot downward towards the floor. Keep your heel in contact with the floor the entire time.

Heel Slides

_____ Reps	_____ Sets	_____X Day	_____ Hold

11 Notes:

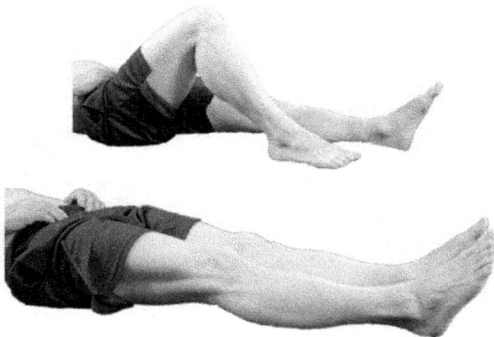

HEEL SLIDES - SUPINE

Lie on your back with knees straight and slide the target heel towards your buttock as you bend your knee. Hold a gentle stretch in this position and then return to original position.

_____ Reps	_____ Sets	_____X Day	_____ Hold

12 Notes:

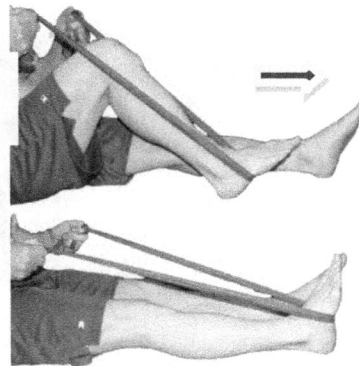

Starting Position

HEEL SLIDES - RESISTED EXTENSION – ELASTIC BAND

Long sit with band around bottom of target foot. Slide the target heel towards your buttock as you bend your knee. Push your foot to straighten knee against resistance to the original position.

Quadriceps (QUAD) / Knee Extension

	_____ Reps _____ Sets _____ X Day _____ Hold
13	**Notes:**

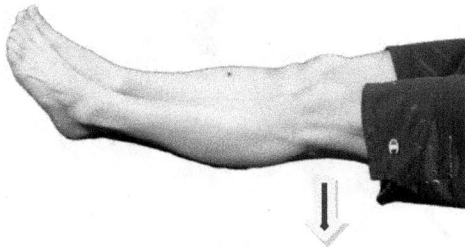

QUAD SET –ISOMETRIC

Tighten your top thigh muscle as you attempt to press the back of your knee downward towards the table. Hold 5-10 seconds. Repeat.

	_____ Reps _____ Sets _____ X Day _____ Hold
14	**Notes:**

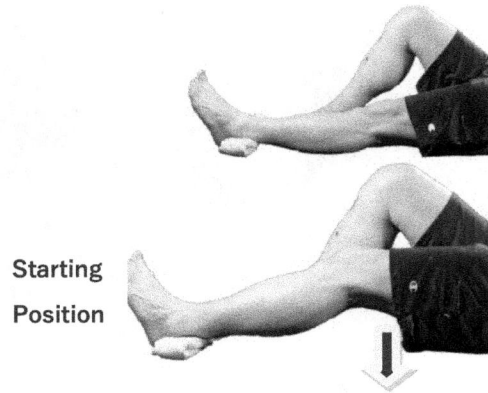

Starting Position

QUAD SET WITH TOWEL UNDER HEEL - ISOMETRIC

Lying or sitting with a small towel roll under your ankle, tighten your top thigh muscle to press the back of your knee downward towards the ground. Hold 5-10 seconds. Repeat.

	_____ Reps _____ Sets _____ X Day _____ Hold
15	**Notes:**

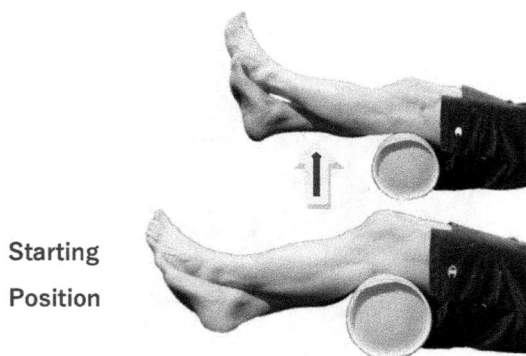

Starting Position

SHORT ARC QUAD (SAQ) – SELF ASSISTED

Place a rolled-up towel or other rounded object under your knee. Hook one foot under the other to assist the affected leg. Slowly straighten your knee as your raise up your foot tightening the top thigh muscle.

	_____ Reps _____ Sets _____ X Day _____ Hold
16	**Notes:**

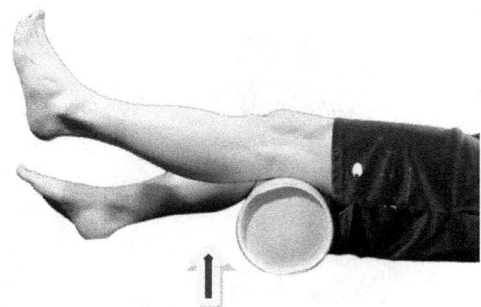

SHORT ARC QUAD - (SAQ) - Can add ankle weight

Place a rolled-up towel or object under your knee and slowly straighten your knee as your raise up your foot tightening the top thigh muscle. Flex your foot to increase the stretch.

	_____ Reps _____ Sets _____ X Day _____ Hold
17	Notes:

KNEE EXTENSION - SELF ASSISTED

In a seated position, place the unaffected leg under the target leg. Use the unaffected leg to assist the target leg up to a straightened knee position.

	_____ Reps _____ Sets _____ X Day _____ Hold
18	Notes:

PARTIAL ARC QUAD - LOW SEAT - Can add ankle weight

Sit with your knee in a semi bent position and your heel touching the ground and then slowly straighten your knee as you raise your foot upwards as shown. Lower your foot back down slowly controlling the muscle until your heel touches the ground and then repeat.

	_____ Reps _____ Sets _____ X Day _____ Hold
19	Notes:

LONG ARC QUAD (LAQ) – LOW SEAT (90 deg)

Sit with your knee in a bent position and then tighten the quadricep. Slowly straighten your knee as you raise your foot upwards as shown. Lower your foot back down to original bent knee position slowly controlling the muscle and then repeat.

	_____ Reps _____ Sets _____ X Day _____ Hold
20	Notes:

LONG ARC QUAD (LAQ) – LOW SEAT - ANKLE WEIGHTS

Attach and ankle weight. Sit with your knee in a bent position and then tighten the quadricep. Slowly straighten your knee as you raise your foot upwards as shown. Lower your foot back down to original bent knee position slowly controlling the muscle - repeat.

_____ Reps _____ Sets _____ X Day _____ Hold		

21 — Notes:

LONG ARC QUAD (LAQ) - HIGH SEAT

Sit with your knee in a bent position and then tighten the quadricep. Slowly straighten your knee as you raise your foot upwards as shown. Lower your foot back down to original bent knee position slowly controlling the muscle and then repeat.

_____ Reps _____ Sets _____ X Day _____ Hold

22 — Notes:

LONG ARC QUAD (LAQ) - HIGH SEAT - ANKLE WEIGHTS

Attach and ankle weight. Sit with your knee in a bent position and then tighten the quadricep. Slowly straighten your knee as you raise your foot upwards as shown. Lower your foot back down to original bent knee position slowly controlling the muscle and then repeat.

_____ Reps _____ Sets _____ X Day _____ Hold

23 — Notes:

LONG ARC QUAD - ELASTIC BAND – HANDHELD

Attach a looped elastic band to your ankle and to the opposite foot or hold with your hand. Sit with your knee in a bent position and then tighten the quadricep. Draw your lower leg upwards to a straighten knee position while your other foot or hand secures the band. Lower your foot back down to original bent knee position slowly controlling the muscle and then repeat.

_____ Reps _____ Sets _____ X Day _____ Hold

24 — Notes:

LONG ARC QUAD - ELASTIC BAND

Attach a looped elastic band to your ankle and to a steady object behind you. Sit with your knee in a bent position and then tighten the quadricep. Draw your lower leg upwards to a straightened knee position. Lower your foot back down to original bent knee position slowly controlling the muscle and then repeat.

Hamstrings

	_____ Reps _____ Sets _____ X Day _____ Hold
25	**Notes:**

HAMSTRING CURLS - PRONE - ASSISTED

Lie face down and hook one foot under the other to assist the affected leg. Bend the target leg with the assistance of your unaffected leg.

	_____ Reps _____ Sets _____ X Day _____ Hold
26	**Notes:**

HAMSTRING CURLS - PRONE

Lie face down and slowly bend your knee as you bring your foot towards your buttock.

	_____ Reps _____ Sets _____ X Day _____ Hold
27	**Notes:**

HAMSTRING CURLS - - PRONE - WEIGHTS

Attach and ankle weight. Lie face down and slowly bend your knee as you bring your foot towards your buttock.

	_____ Reps _____ Sets _____ X Day _____ Hold
28	**Notes:**

HAMSTRING CURLS – PRONE - ELASTIC BAND

Attach an elastic band around your foot and opposite ankle as shown. While lying face down, slowly bend your target knee as you bring your foot towards your buttock. Keep your other foot on the floor to fixate the band.

	_____ Reps _____ Sets _____X Day _____Hold
29	**Notes:**

HAMSTRING CURLS – ELASTIC BAND

Sit and use an elastic band secured to a steady object and the other end attached to your ankle. Bend your knee and draw back your foot.

	_____ Reps _____ Sets _____X Day _____Hold
30	**Notes:**

HAMSTRING CURLS – ELASTIC BAND - 2

Attach a looped elastic band to your ankle and to the opposite foot while one leg is propped on stool or another raised object. Draw your lower leg downwards to a bent knee position while your other ankle anchors the band on the chair.

	_____ Reps _____ Sets _____X Day _____Hold
31	**Notes:**

HAMSTRING CURLS ON BALL – can add ankle weight.

Lie prone on an exercise ball as shown. Slowly bend your knee as you bring your foot towards your buttock.

	_____ Reps _____ Sets _____X Day _____Hold
32	**Notes:** **Advanced**

Starting Position

HAMSTRING CURLS - SINGLE LEG - EXERCISE BALL

Lie on the floor and place your heel on an exercise ball.
Lift your buttocks and then bend your knees to draw the ball towards your buttocks. Keep your buttocks elevated off the floor the entire time.

Hip Flexion

	_____ Reps _____ Sets _____ X Day _____ Hold
33	**Notes:**

HIP FLEXION ISOMETRIC

Lie on your back, lift up your knee and press it into your hand. Hold. Return to the original position and repeat.

HIP FLEXION ISOMETRIC - ALTERNATING
Lie on your back, lift up your knee and press it into your hand. Hold. Return to the original position and repeat on the other side.

	_____ Reps _____ Sets _____ X Day _____ Hold
34	**Notes:**

HIP FLEXION ISOMETRIC BILATERAL

Lie on your back, lift up your knees and press them into your hands. Hold. Return to the original position and repeat.

	_____ Reps _____ Sets _____ X Day _____ Hold
35	**Notes:**

HIP FLEXION – ISOMETRIC - Can use towel roll for comfort

While standing in front of a wall, draw your knee forward and press it into the wall. Place a folded towel between your knee and the wall for comfort if needed.

	_____ Reps _____ Sets _____ X Day _____ Hold
36	**Notes:**

STRAIGHT LEG RAISE (SLR)

Lie on your back, tighten the quad of the target leg and lift up with a straight knee. Keep the opposite knee bent with the foot planted on the ground. (see #37 for starting position)

	_____ Reps _____ Sets _____X Day _____Hold
37	**Notes:**

Starting

Position

STRAIGHT LEG RAISE (SLR) – ANKLE WEIGHTS

Attach ankle weights. Lie on your back and lift up your leg with a straight knee. Keep the opposite knee bent with the foot planted on the ground

	_____ Reps _____ Sets _____X Day _____Hold
38	**Notes:**

STRAIGHT LEG RAISE (SLR) - ELASTIC BAND

Lie on your back with an elastic band looped around your ankles, lift the target leg upwards.

	_____ Reps _____ Sets _____X Day _____Hold
39	**Notes:**

SEATED MARCHING - can add ankle weights for resistance

Sit in a chair and move a knee upward, set it back down and then alternate to the other side

	_____ Reps _____ Sets _____X Day _____Hold
40	**Notes:**

SEATED MARCHING - ELASTIC BAND

Sit in a chair with an elastic band wrapped around your thighs. Move a knee upward, set it back down and then alternate to the other side.

Hip Extension

	_____ Reps _____ Sets _____X Day _____Hold		_____ Reps _____ Sets _____X Day _____Hold
41	**Notes:**	**42**	**Notes:**

HIP EXTENSION - PRONE

Lie face down with your knee straight and slowly lift up leg off the ground. Maintain a straight knee the entire time.

HIP EXTENSION – PRONE – ANKLE WEIGHTS

Attach ankle weights. Lie face down with your knee straight and slowly lift up leg off the ground. Maintain a straight knee the entire time.

	_____ Reps _____ Sets _____X Day _____Hold		_____ Reps _____ Sets _____X Day _____Hold
43	**Notes:**	**44**	**Notes:**

HIP EXTENSION – PRONE – ELASTIC BAND

Lie on your stomach with an elastic band looped around your ankles and lift the targeted leg upwards. Maintain a straight knee the entire time.

HIP EXTENSION – QUADRUPED with or without ankle weights

Start in a crawl position and then raise your leg up behind you as shown. Keep your knee bent at 90 degrees the entire time.

Hip Abduction (ABD)

45	_____ Reps _____ Sets _____ X Day _____ Hold		
	Notes:		

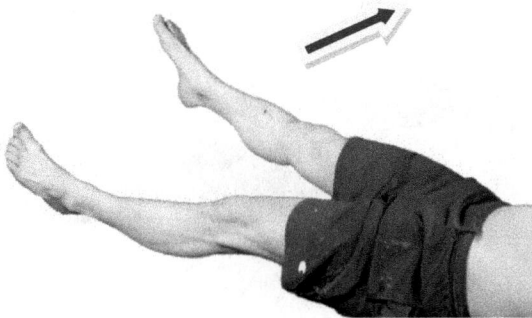

HIP ABDUCTION - SUPINE

Lie on your back and slowly bring your leg out to the side. Return to original position and repeat. Keep your knee straight the entire time.

46	_____ Reps _____ Sets _____ X Day _____ Hold		
	Notes:		

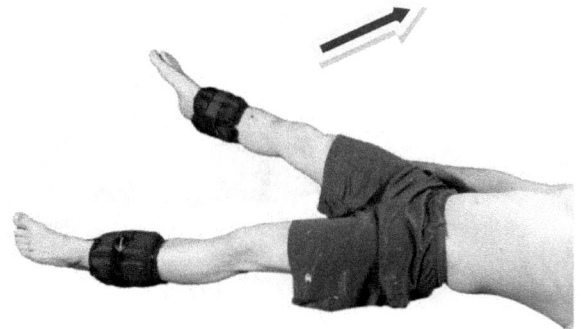

HIP ABDUCTION - SUPINE – ANKLE WEIGHTS

Attach and weights. Lie on your back and slowly bring your leg up slightly and then out to the side. Return to original position and repeat. Keep your knee straight the entire time.

47	_____ Reps _____ Sets _____ X Day _____ Hold		
	Notes:		

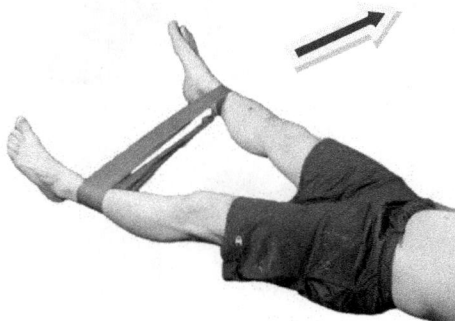

HIP ABDUCTION – SUPINE - ELASTIC BAND

Lie on your back and slowly bring your leg out to the side. Return to original position and repeat. Keep your knee straight the entire time.

48	_____ Reps _____ Sets _____ X Day _____ Hold		
	Notes:		

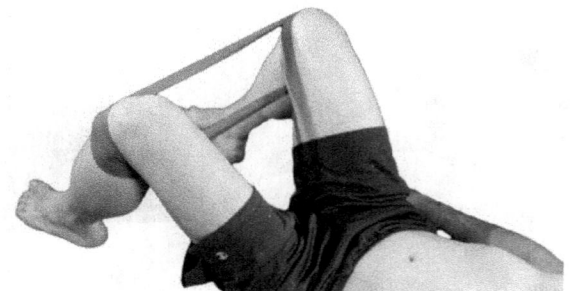

HIP ABDUCTION / CLAMS– SUPINE - ELASTIC BAND

Lie down on your back with your knees bent. Place an elastic band around your knees and then draw your knees apart. Return to original position and repeat.

	_____ Reps _____ Sets _____ X Day _____ Hold		_____ Reps _____ Sets _____ X Day _____ Hold
49	**Notes:**	**50**	**Notes:**

MODIFIED HIP ABDUCTION – SIDELYING can add weights

Lie on your side and slowly lift up your top leg to the side. The bottom leg can be bent to stabilize your body. Keep your knee straight and maintain your toes pointed forward the entire time. Keep your leg in-line with your body. Return to original position and repeat.

HIP ABDUCTION – SIDELYING

Lie on your side and slowly lift up your top leg to the side. Keep your knee straight and maintain your toes pointed forward the entire time. Keep your leg in-line with your body. Return to original position and repeat.

	_____ Reps _____ Sets _____ X Day _____ Hold		_____ Reps _____ Sets _____ X Day _____ Hold
51	**Notes:**	**52**	**Notes:**

HIP ABDUCTION – SIDELYING - WEIGHTS

Attach ankle weights. Lie on your side and slowly lift up your top leg to the side. Keep your knee straight and maintain your toes pointed forward the entire time. Keep your leg in-line with your body. Return to original position and repeat.

HIP ABDUCTION – SIDELYING - ELASTIC BAND

Lie on your side with an elastic band looped around your ankles. Lift the top leg upwards keeping your knee straight and maintaining your toes pointed forward the entire time. Keep your leg in-line with your body. Return to original position and repeat.

	_____ Reps _____ Sets _____ X Day _____ Hold
53	**Notes:**

Starting
Position

CLAM SHELLS

Lie on your side with your knees bent, draw up the top knee while keeping contact of your feet together.
Do not let your pelvis roll back during the lifting movement.

	_____ Reps _____ Sets _____ X Day _____ Hold
54	**Notes:**

Starting
Position

SIDELYING CLAM - ELASTIC BAND

Lie on your side with your knees bent and an elastic band wrapped around your knees, draw up the top knee while keeping contact of your feet together as shown. Do not let your pelvis roll back during the lifting movement.

	_____ Reps _____ Sets _____ X Day _____ Hold
55	**Notes:**

Starting
Position

HIP ABDUCTION - FIRE HYDRANT - QUADRUPED

Start in a crawl position and raise your leg out to the side as shown. Maintain a straight upper and mid back.

	_____ Reps _____ Sets _____ X Day _____ Hold
56	**Notes:**

Starting
Position

HIP ABDUCTION - FIRE HYDRANT – QUADRUPED - ELASTIC BAND

Start in a crawl position with an elastic band around your thighs. Raise your leg out to the side as shown. Maintain a straight upper and mid back.

	_____ Reps _____ Sets _____X Day _____Hold		_____ Reps _____ Sets _____X Day _____Hold
57	**Notes:**	**58**	**Notes:**

HIP ABDUCTION - SEATED - STRAIGHT LEG

Sit close to the edge of a chair with your target leg straight at the knee. Move your target leg to the side lifting slightly off the ground and then return to straight ahead.. You can slide your heel across the floor as you move and then return to straight ahead if unable to lift. Maintain your toes pointed up the entire time.

HIP ABDUCTION - SEATED - STRAIGHT LEG – ANKLE WEIGHT

Attach an ankle weight. Sit close to the edge of a chair with your target leg straight at the knee. Move your target leg to the side lifting slightly off the ground and then return to straight ahead. Maintain your toes pointed up the entire time.

	_____ Reps _____ Sets _____X Day _____Hold		_____ Reps _____ Sets _____X Day _____Hold
59	**Notes:**	**60**	**Notes:**

HIP ABDUCTION - SINGLE- SEATED

Sit close to the edge of a chair with knees bent and both feet on the floor. Move your target knee out to the side as shown and then return to straight ahead. Maintain contact of your feet on the floor the entire time.

HIP ABDUCTION - SINGLE- SEATED – ELASTIC BAND

With band tied around the thighs, sit close to the edge of a chair with knees bent and both feet on the floor. Move your target knee out to the side as shown and then return to straight ahead. Maintain contact of your feet on the floor the entire time.tact of your feet on the floor the entire time.

	_____ Reps _____ Sets _____ X Day _____ Hold
61	**Notes:**

HIP ABDUCTION - BILATERAL- SEATED

Sit close to the edge of a chair with knees bent and both feet on the floor. Move your knees out to the side as shown and then return to straight ahead. Maintain contact of your feet on the floor the entire time.

	_____ Reps _____ Sets _____ X Day _____ Hold
62	**Notes:**

HIP ABDUCTION - BILATERAL- SEATED - ELASTIC BAND

Sit close to the edge of a chair with an elastic band wrapped around your knees. Move both knees to the sides to separate your legs. Keep contact of your feet on the floor the entire time.

Hip Adduction (ADD)

	_____ Reps _____ Sets _____ X Day _____ Hold
63	**Notes:**

HIP ADDUCTION SQUEEZE – SUPINE – KNEES BENT

Lie on your back with legs bent and place a rolled up towel, ball or pillow between your knees. Press your knees together so that you squeeze the object firmly. Hold, release and repeat.

	_____ Reps _____ Sets _____ X Day _____ Hold
64	**Notes:**

HIP ADDUCTION SQUEEZE – SUPINE – LEGS STRAIGHT

Lie on your back and place a rolled up towel, ball or pillow between your knees. Squeeze the object with your knees. Hold, release and repeat.

	_____ Reps _____ Sets _____X Day _____Hold
65	**Notes:**

HIP ADDUCTION - SIDELYING

Lie on your side, slowly lift up your bottom leg towards the ceiling. Keep your knee straight the entire time. Your top leg should be bent at the knee and your foot planted on the ground supporting your body.

	_____ Reps _____ Sets _____X Day _____Hold
66	**Notes:**

BALL SQUEEZE - SEATED

Sit and place a rolled-up towel, ball or pillow between your knees and squeeze the object firmly. Hold, release and repeat.

Hip Internal Rotation (IR)

	_____ Reps _____ Sets _____X Day _____Hold
67	**Notes:**

INTERNAL ROTATION - HEEL SQUEEZE - ISOMETRIC

Lie face down, spead your knees apart and press your heels together. Hold, release and repeat.

	_____ Reps _____ Sets _____X Day _____Hold
68	**Notes:**

HIP INTERNAL ROTATION - SUPINE

Lie on your back with your knees straight, roll your hip in so that your toes point inward. Be sure that your knee cap faces inward as well.

_____ Reps _____ Sets _____X Day _____Hold

69 | Notes:

Starting
Position

REVERSE CLAMS - SIDELYING

Lie on your side with your knees bent and raise your top foot towards the ceiling while keeping contact of your knees together. Lower back down to original position. Do not let your pelvis roll forward during the lifting movement.

_____ Reps _____ Sets _____X Day _____Hold

70 | Notes:

Starting Position

REVERSE CLAMS - SIDELYING - ELASTIC BAND

Lie on your side with your knees bent and an elastic band around your ankles. Raise your top foot towards the ceiling while keeping contact of your knees together. Lower back down to original position. Do not let your pelvis roll forward during the lifting movement.

_____ Reps _____ Sets _____X Day _____Hold

71 | Notes:

HIP INTERNAL ROTATION - SEATED

Sit on a chair with your legs spread apart and feet planted on the ground. Use your hand on the inside of your knee to resist the movement inward.

_____ Reps _____ Sets _____X Day _____Hold

72 | Notes:

HIP INTERNAL ROTATION - ELASTIC BAND - High chair

Attach one end of an elastic band at your ankle and the other to a sturdy object. Pull away from your other leg while keeping your thigh from moving.

Hip External Rotation (ER)

	_____ Reps _____ Sets _____X Day _____Hold		_____ Reps _____ Sets _____X Day _____Hold
73	Notes:	74	Notes:

HIP EXTERNAL ROTATION - SUPINE

Lie on your back with your knees straight and roll your hip out so that your toes point outward. Be sure that your knee cap faces outward as well.

HIP EXTERNAL ROTATION - ELASTIC BAND

Sit and use an elastic band secured to a steady object and the other end attached to your ankle from the side.
Pull towards your other leg while keeping your thigh from moving across the table.

Bilateral Hip Rotation

	_____ Reps _____ Sets _____X Day _____Hold		_____ Reps _____ Sets _____X Day _____Hold
75	Notes:	76	Notes:

HIP ROTATIONS – BILATERAL - SIDELYING

Lie on your side in fetal position with knees and hips bent.
Slowly raise up both lower legs and feet as shown.
Your feet and knees should be touching the entire time.

HIP ROTATION - SEATED - BALL and ELASTIC BAND – High chair

Sit and place a rolled-up towel, ball or pillow between your knees and an elastic band around your ankles. Squeeze the ball, sustain and hold. Next, pull the band as you move your feet apart from each other.

Leg Press

_____ Reps _____ Sets _____ X Day _____ Hold		_____ Reps _____ Sets _____ X Day _____ Hold
77 Notes:		**78** Notes:

Starting
Position

PRESS – BILATERAL – ELASTIC BAND

Lie on back put elastic band on bottom of both feet. Start with knees bent and push with feet to straighten both legs.

PRESS – SINGLE LEG – ELASTIC BAND

Lie on back put elastic band on bottom of one foot. Start with knees bent and push with foot to straighten leg.

Hip Hikes (Gluteus Medius)

_____ Reps _____ Sets _____ X Day _____ Hold		_____ Reps _____ Sets _____ X Day _____ Hold
79 Notes:		**80** Notes:

HIP HIKE - STANDING on Step or Pad

Stand with one foot on a step or pad and the other hanging off as shown. Raise and lower the side of your pelvis that is hanging off the edge.

HIP HIKE – KNEELING on towel or pad

Kneel on both knees with one knee on a folded towel or pad. Raise and lower the side of your pelvis that is not on the towel/pad.

Glutes (Glute Max)

	_____ Reps _____ Sets ____X Day ____Hold		_____ Reps _____ Sets ____X Day ____Hold
81	**Notes:**	**82**	**Notes:**

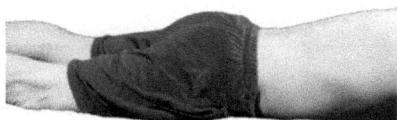

GLUTE SETS - PRONE

Lie face down, squeeze your buttocks and hold. Repeat.

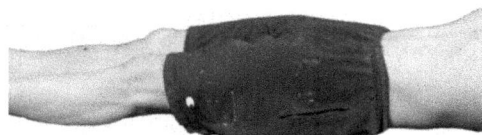

GLUTE SET - SUPINE

Lie on your back, squeeze your buttocks and hold. Repeat.

	_____ Reps _____ Sets ____X Day ____Hold		_____ Reps _____ Sets ____X Day ____Hold
83	**Notes:**	**84**	**Notes:**

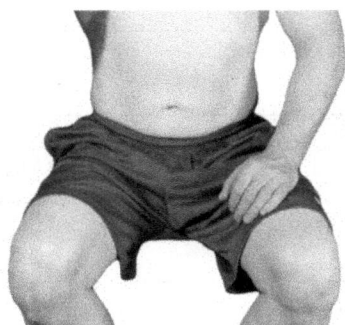

GLUTE SQUEEZE - SITTING

While sitting, squeeze your buttocks and hold. Repeat.

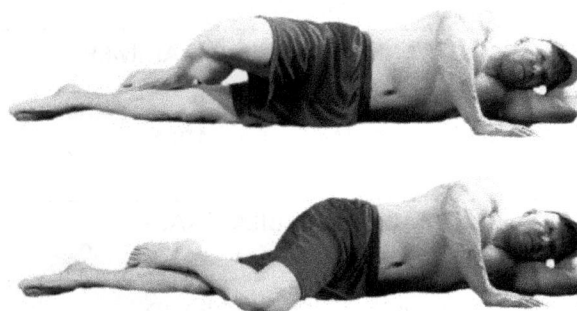

GLUTE SCULPT (MAX/MEDIUS)

Lie on your side leaning towards your stomach. Bend leg on target side, raise up and hold.

EXERCISE Upper Extremity Strengthening and Range of Motion	EXERCISE NUMBER	NOTES
ELBOW FLEXION EXTENSION - SUPINE	1	
ELBOW FLEXION / EXTENSION - GRAVITY ELIMINATED	2	
BICEPS CURLS – ALTERNATING	3	
BICEPS CURL - SELF FIXATION – ELASTIC BAND	4	
SEATED BICEPS CURLS - ALTERNATING	5	
SEATED BICEPS CURLS - BILATERAL	6	
CONCENTRATION CURLS – SITTING	7	
PREACHER CURL ON BALL	8	
BICEPS CURLS	9	
BICEPS CURLS - RADIOBRACHIALIS - HAMMER CURL	10	
BICEPS CURLS - BRACHIALIS	11	
BICEPS CURLS – ROTATE OUTWARD	12	
BICEPS CURLS – ONE ARM - ELASTIC BAND	13	
BICEPS CURLS – BILATERAL - ELASTIC BAND	14	
BICEPS CURLS - RADIOBRACHIALIS - HAMMER CURL – ONE ARM - ELASTIC BAND	15	
BICEPS CURLS - RADIOBRACHIALIS - HAMMER CURL – BILATERAL - ELASTIC BAND	16	
BICEPS CURLS – BRACHIALIS - ONE ARM - ELASTIC BAND	17	
BICEPS CURL – BRACHIALIS – BILATERAL - ELASTIC BAND	18	
TRICEPS - SELF FIXATION - ELASTIC BAND	19	
OVERHEAD TRICEPS - SELF FIXATION –SEATED OR STANDING - ELASTIC BAND	20	
TRICEP EXTENSION – SITTING OR STANDING - WEIGHT	21	
TRICEP EXTENSION – SITTING OR STANDING – BILATERAL - WEIGHT	22	
ELBOW EXTENSION - BALL	23	

EXERCISE Upper Extremity Strengthening and Range of Motion	EXERCISE NUMBER	NOTES
ELBOW EXTENSION - SKULL CRUSHER - BALL	24	
TRICEPS - ELASTIC BAND	25	
TRICEPS - BENT OVER	26	
CHAIR DIPS / PUSH UPS	27	
DIPS OFF CHAIR	28	
PENDULUM SHOULDER FORWARD/BACK	29	
PENDULUM SHOULDER – SIDE TO SIDE	30	
PENDULUM SHOULDER CIRCLES	31	
PENDULUMS - SUPINE	32	
ISOMETRIC FLEXION	33	
SHOULDER FLEXION – SIDELYING	34	
FLEXION – SUPINE - SINGLE OR BILATERAL	35	
FLEXION – SUPINE – SINGLE OR BILATERAL - WEIGHT	36	
FLEXION – SUPINE - DOWEL	37	
FLEXION – SUPINE - DOWEL - Weight	38	
FLEXION - SELF FIXATION – ELASTIC BAND	39	
FLEXION – ELASTIC BAND	40	
FLEXION - STANDING - PALMS DOWN / OVERHAND DOWEL	41	
FLEXION - STANDING - PALMS UP / UNDERHAND DOWEL	42	
FLEXION – PALMS FACING INWARD	43	
FLEXION – PALMS DOWN	44	
V RAISE	45	
V RAISE – WEIGHTS	46	
MILITARY PRESS – DOWEL	47	
MILITARY PRESS - FREE WEIGHTS	48	

EXERCISE Upper Extremity Strengthening and Range of Motion	EXERCISE NUMBER	NOTES
ISOMETRIC EXTENSION	49	
PRONE EXTENSION - EXERCISE BALL	50	
SHOULDER EXTENSION - STANDING	51	
SHOULDER EXTENSION - STANDING - WEIGHTS	52	
EXTENSION – STANDING – DOWEL	53	
EXTENSION - SELF FIXATION - ELASTIC BAND	54	
EXTENSION - ELASTIC BAND	55	
EXTENSION - BILATERAL - ELASTIC BAND	56	
INTERNAL ROTATION – ISOMETRIC	57	
INTERNAL ROTATION - ISOMETRIC- ELEVATED	58	
INTERNAL ROTATION - SIDELYING	59	
INTERNAL ROTATION - ELASTIC BAND	60	
INTERNAL / EXTERNAL ROTATION - STANDING – DOWEL	61	
INTERNAL ROTATION – DOWEL	62	
EXTERNAL ROTATION - ISOMETRIC	63	
EXTERNAL ROTATION - ISOMETRIC – ELEVATED	64	
EXTERNAL ROTATION WITH TOWEL - SIDELYING	65	
EXTERNAL ROTATION – 90/90 - WEIGHTS	66	
EXTERNAL ROTATION - BILATERAL - ELASTIC BAND	67	
EXTERNAL ROTATION - ELASTIC BAND	68	
ADDUCTION – ISOMETRIC	69	
ADDUCTION - ELASTIC BAND	70	
ABDUCTION – ISOMETRIC	71	
HORIZONTAL ABDUCTION - DOWEL	72	

EXERCISE Upper Extremity Strengthening and Range of Motion	EXERCISE NUMBER	NOTES
HORIZONTAL ABDUCTION/ADDUCTTION - SUPINE	73	
HORIZONTAL ABDUCTION/ADDUCTTION - SUPINE -WEIGHT	74	
ABDUCTION - SIDELYING	75	
HORIZONTAL ABDUCTION - SIDELYING	76	
ABDUCTION – WEIGHT	77	
ABDUCTION – ELASTIC BAND	78	
HORIZONTAL ABDUCTION – BILATERAL - ELASTIC BAND	79	
90/90 ABDUCTION - WEIGHT	80	
LATERAL RAISES	81	
LATERAL RAISES – LEAN FORWARD	82	
LATERAL RAISES – LEAN FORWARD - ARM ROTATION	83	
FRONTAL RAISE – WEIGHTS	84	
UPRIGHT ROW – WEIGHTS	85	
UPRIGHT ROW – ELASTIC BAND	86	
SHRUGS	87	
SHRUGS - WEIGHTS	88	
SHOULDER ROLLS	89	
SHOULDER ROLLS - WEIGHTS	90	
SCAPULAR RETRACTIONS - BILATERAL	91	
SCAPULAR RETRACTION – SINGLE ARM	92	
ELASTIC BAND SCAPULAR RETRACTIONS WITH MINI SHOULDER EXTENSIONS	93	
PRONE RETRACTION	94	
SCAPULAR PROTRACTION - SUPINE - BILATERAL	95	
SCAPULAR PROTRACTION - SUPINE - WEIGHT	96	

EXERCISE Upper Extremity Strengthening and Range of Motion	EXERCISE NUMBER	NOTES
SCAPULAR PROTRACTION - SUPINE - ELASTIC BAND	97	
SCAPULAR PROTRACTION / TABLE PLANK	98	
CHEST PRESS – SEATED or STANDING - ELASTIC BAND	99	
CHEST PRESS – BALL, FLOOR or BENCH- WEIGHTS	100	
DOWEL PRESS – STANDING	101	
CHEST PRESS – STANDING or SEATED	102	
BENT OVER ROWS	103	
ROWS – PRONE	104	
ROWS - ELASTIC BAND	105	
WIDE ROWS - ELASTIC BAND	106	
LOW ROW – ELASTIC BAND	107	
HIGH ROW – ELASTIC BAND	108	
FLY'S – FLOOR - WEIGHT	109	
FLY'S – BALL or BENCH – WEIGHT	110	
WALL PUSH UPS	111	
WALL PUSH UP - BALL	112	
WALL PUSH UP - Triceps uneven	113	
WALL PUSH UP - Hands inverted	114	
WALL PUSH UP - Narrow	115	
WALL PUSH UP – Wide	116	
PUSH UPS - BALL	117	
PUSH UP - MODIFIED	118	
PUSH UP	119	
PUSH UP -DIAMOND	120	
PUSH UP – MODIFIED - BOSU - UNSTABLE	121	

EXERCISE Upper Extremity Strengthening and Range of Motion	EXERCISE NUMBER	NOTES
PUSH UP – BOSU - UNSTABLE	122	
PUSH UP – MODIFIED – INVERTED BOSU - UNSTABLE	123	
PUSH UP – INVERTED BOSU - UNSTABLE	124	

UPPER EXTREMITY - Range Of Motion > Isometric > Strength

Elbow Flexion/Extension

	_____ Reps _____ Sets _____X Day _____Hold		_____ Reps _____ Sets _____X Day _____Hold
1	Notes:	**2**	Notes:

ELBOW FLEXION EXTENSION - SUPINE

Lie on your back and rest your elbow on a small rolled up towel. Bend at your elbow and then lower back down.

ELBOW FLEXION / EXTENSION - GRAVITY ELIMINATED

Sit and hold your arm up with the help of your other arm. Bend and straighten your elbow.

Elbow Flexion (Biceps)

	_____ Reps _____ Sets _____X Day _____Hold		_____ Reps _____ Sets _____X Day _____Hold
3	Notes:	**4**	Notes:

BICEPS CURLS – ALTERNATING

Bend your elbow and move your forearm upwards. As you lower back down, begin bending the opposite elbow upwards.

BICEPS CURL - SELF FIXATION – ELASTIC BAND

Sit and hold an elastic band with one hand. Hold the other end of elastic band with the opposite hand and fixate hand on your knee. Slowly draw up your hand by bending at the elbow. Return to starting position and repeat.

*Can increase resistance by doubling band as shown.

	_____ Reps _____ Sets _____X Day _____Hold		_____ Reps _____ Sets _____X Day _____Hold
5	Notes:	**6**	Notes:

SEATED BICEPS CURLS - ALTERNATING

Sit in a chair and hold free weights on each thigh. Lift one side while bending at the elbow and squeezing bicep muscle. Perform on one side and then alternate to the other side.

SEATED BICEPS CURLS - BILATERAL

Sit in a chair and hold free weights on each thigh. Lift both sides while bending at the elbows and squeezing bicep muscles. Lower back down and repeat.

	_____ Reps _____ Sets _____X Day _____Hold		_____ Reps _____ Sets _____X Day _____Hold
7	Notes:	**8**	Notes:

CONCENTRATION CURLS – SITTING

Sit in a chair, lean slightly forward and hold a free weight with arm straight with elbow on inside of thigh. Bend elbow squeezing bicep muscle. Lower back down - repeat.

Starting Position

PREACHER CURL ON BALL

Lie on stomach over ball in crawling position. Hold weights in both hands with back of arms against ball. Lift both sides while bending at the elbows and squeezing bicep muscles. Lower back down - repeat.

	_____ Reps _____ Sets _____X Day _____Hold
9	Notes:

BICEPS CURLS

Holding weights and keeping your arm at your side, draw up your hand by bending at the elbow squeezing bicep muscle. Keep your palm face up the entire time. Can perform set on one side and then other or alternate arms.

	_____ Reps _____ Sets _____X Day _____Hold
10	Notes:

BICEPS CURLS - RADIOBRACHIALIS - HAMMER CURL

Holding weights and keeping your arm at your side, draw up your hand by bending at the elbow squeezing bicep muscle. Keep your wrist in a neutral position as shown above the entire time. Can perform set on one side and then other or alternate arms.

	_____ Reps _____ Sets _____X Day _____Hold
11	Notes:

BICEPS CURLS - BRACHIALIS

Holding weights and keeping your arm at your side, draw up your hand by bending at the elbow squeezing bicep muscle. Keep your palm face down the entire time. Can perform set on one side and then other or alternate arms.

	_____ Reps _____ Sets _____X Day ____Hold
12	Notes:

BICEPS CURLS – ROTATE OUTWARD

Holding weights and keeping your arm at your side, draw up your hand by bending at the elbow squeezing bicep muscle. Keep your palm face up the entire time. You can do this one arm at a time or bilateral.

13	_____ Reps _____ Sets _____X Day _____Hold Notes:

BICEPS CURLS – ONE ARM - ELASTIC BAND

In a standing position, step on the band with one leg. Keep your arm at your side holding an elastic band and draw up your hand by bending at the elbow squeezing bicep muscle. Keep your palm face up the entire time.

14	_____ Reps _____ Sets _____X Day _____Hold Notes:

BICEPS CURLS – BILATERAL - ELASTIC BAND

In a standing position, step on the band with both feet, shoulder width apart. Keep your arms at your side holding an elastic band and draw up your hands by bending at the elbows squeezing bicep muscles. Keep your palms facing upward the entire time.

15	_____ Reps _____ Sets _____X Day _____Hold Notes:

BICEPS CURLS - RADIOBRACHIALIS - HAMMER CURL – ONE ARM - ELASTIC BAND

In a standing position, step on the band with one leg. Keep your arm at your side holding an elastic band and draw up your hand by bending at the elbow squeezing bicep muscle. Keep your palm facing inward the entire time.

16	_____ Reps _____ Sets _____X Day _____Hold Notes:

BICEPS CURLS - RADIOBRACHIALIS - HAMMER CURL – BILATERAL - ELASTIC BAND

In a standing position, step on the band with both feet, shoulder width apart. Keep your arms at your side holding an elastic band and draw up your hands by bending at the elbows squeezing bicep muscles. Keep your palms facing inward the entire time.

	_____ Reps _____ Sets _____ X Day _____ Hold		_____ Reps _____ Sets _____ X Day _____ Hold
17	**Notes:**	**18**	**Notes:**

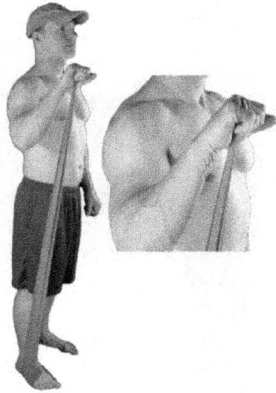

BICEPS CURLS – BRACHIALIS - ONE ARM - ELASTIC BAND

In a standing position, step on the band with one leg. Keep your arm at your side holding an elastic band and draw up your hand by bending at the elbow squeezing bicep muscle. Keep your palm face down the entire time.

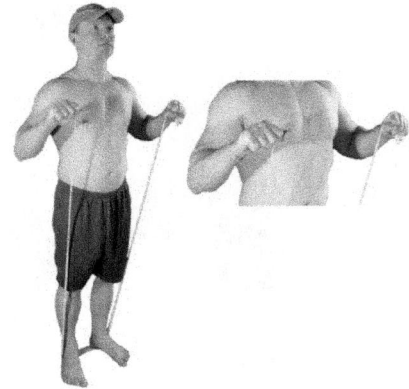

BICEPS CURL – BRACHIALIS – BILATERAL - ELASTIC BAND

In a standing position, step on the band with both feet, shoulder width apart. Keep your arms at your side holding an elastic band and draw up your hands by bending at the elbows squeezing bicep muscles. Keep your palms facing downward the entire time.

Elbow Extension (Triceps)

	_____ Reps _____ Sets _____ X Day _____ Hold		_____ Reps _____ Sets _____ X Day _____ Hold
19	**Notes:**	**20**	**Notes:**

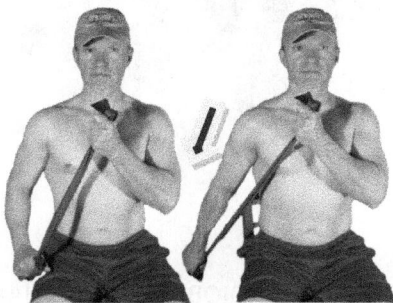

TRICEPS - SELF FIXATION - ELASTIC BAND

Hold an elastic band across your chest with the unaffected arm. Pull the band downward with the other arm so that the elbow goes from a bent position to a straightened position as shown.

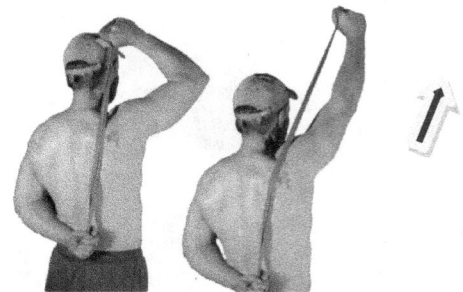

OVERHEAD TRICEPS - SELF FIXATION –SEATED OR STANDING - ELASTIC BAND

Hold an elastic band with one arm fixated behind back as shown and other hand behind head. Extend elbow with arm overhead and return to starting position.

_____ Reps _____ Sets _____ X Day _____ Hold	_____ Reps _____ Sets _____ X Day _____ Hold
21 Notes:	**22** Notes:

TRICEP EXTENSION – SITTING OR STANDING - WEIGHT

Start with hand behind head holding free weight. Extend your elbow as shown. Maintain your upper arm in an upward direction and only bend and straighten at your elbow.
*Can hold the triceps area with opposite arm to stabilize.

TRICEP EXTENSION – SITTING OR STANDING – BILATERAL - WEIGHT

Start with hands behind head holding free weight Extend your elbows while holding a free weight in both hands. Maintain your upper arms in an upward direction and only bend and straighten at your elbows.

_____ Reps _____ Sets _____ X Day _____ Hold	_____ Reps _____ Sets _____ X Day _____ Hold
23 Notes:	**24** Notes:

ELBOW EXTENSION - BALL

Lie on your back on ball. Extend your elbow as shown while holding a free weight in each hand. Maintain your upper arms in an upward direction and only bend and straighten at your elbows.

ELBOW EXTENSION - SKULL CRUSHER - BALL

Lie on your back on ball with a free weight in each hand. Bend your elbows to lower the weight towards the side of your head and then extend arms straight up towards the ceiling.

	_____ Reps _____ Sets _____ X Day _____ Hold		_____ Reps _____ Sets _____ X Day _____ Hold
25	**Notes:**	**26**	**Notes:**

TRICEPS - ELASTIC BAND

Fixate the band at top of door. Start with your elbow bent and holding an elastic band as shown. Pull the elastic band downward as you extend your elbow. Keep your elbow by your side the entire time.

TRICEPS - BENT OVER

Stand and bend over with either support or placing your unaffected arm on thigh for support. With your targeted arm and elbow at your side, extend your elbow as you straighten your arm as shown. Keep your elbow at your side and back flat the entire time.

	_____ Reps _____ Sets _____ X Day _____ Hold		_____ Reps _____ Sets _____ X Day _____ Hold
27	**Notes:**	**28**	**Notes:**

CHAIR DIPS / PUSH UPS

While sitting in a chair with arm rests, push yourself upawards so that you lift your buttocks of the chair and then lower down controlled back to normal seated position. *If you are unable to lift yourself up, you can perform "pressure releases" so that you simply push to take some weight off your buttocks.

DIPS OFF CHAIR

Push yourself up to a straight elbow position as shown. Then lower your buttocks down towards the floor by bending your elbows.

Shoulder PENDULUMS

	_____ Reps _____ Sets _____ X Day _____ Hold		_____ Reps _____ Sets _____ X Day _____ Hold
29	Notes:	**30**	Notes:

PENDULUM SHOULDER FORWARD/BACK

Shift your body weight forward then back to allow your injured arm to swing forward and back freely. Your affected arm should be fully relaxed.

PENDULUM SHOULDER – SIDE TO SIDE

Shift your body weight side to side to allow your injured arm to swing side to side freely. Your affected arm should be fully relaxed.

	_____ Reps _____ Sets _____ X Day _____ Hold		_____ Reps _____ Sets _____ X Day _____ Hold
31	Notes:	**32**	Notes:

PENDULUM SHOULDER CIRCLES
Shift your body weight in circles to allow your injured arm to swing in circles freely. Your injured arm should be fully relaxed.
REVERSE PENDULUM SHOULDER CIRCLES
Shift your body weight into reverse circles to allow your injured arm to swing in circles freely. Your injured arm should be fully relaxed.

PENDULUMS - SUPINE

Lie on your back and straighten your arm towards the ceiling. Move your arm in small circles in a clockwise motion. After a few seconds, reverse the direction to a counterclockwise motion. Change directions every few seconds.

Shoulder Flexion

_____ Reps _____ Sets _____X Day _____Hold	_____ Reps _____ Sets _____X Day _____Hold
33 Notes:	**34** Notes:

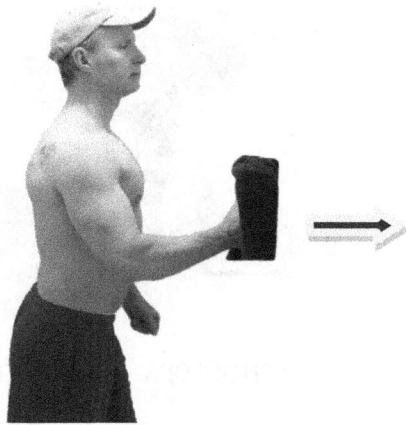

ISOMETRIC FLEXION - Can use towel roll for comfort

Gently push your fist forward into a wall with your elbow bent. Hold for 5-10 seconds. Repeat.

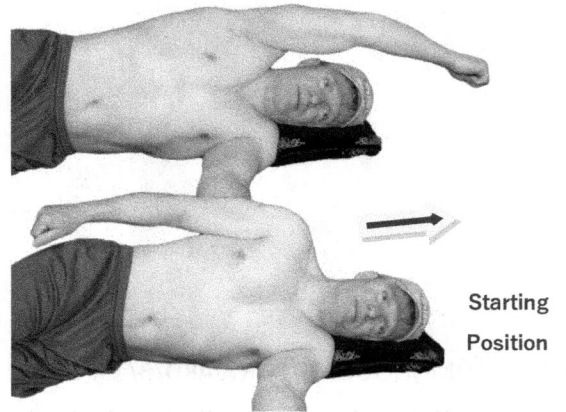

Starting Position

SHOULDER FLEXION – SIDELYING - Can add weight

Lie on your side with arm at your side. Slowly raise the arm forward towards overhead and in front of your body.

_____ Reps _____ Sets _____X Day _____Hold	_____ Reps _____ Sets _____X Day _____Hold
35 Notes:	**36** Notes:

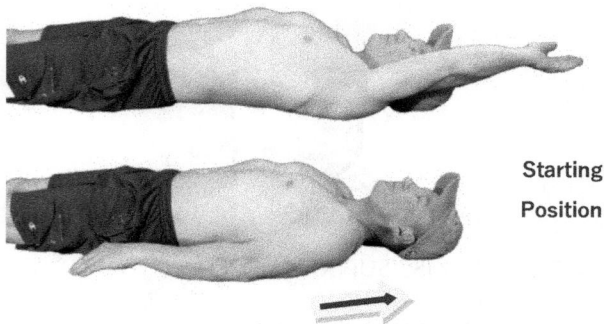

Starting Position

FLEXION – SUPINE - SINGLE OR BILATERAL

Lie on your back with your arm at your side. Slowly raise arm up and forward towards overhead.

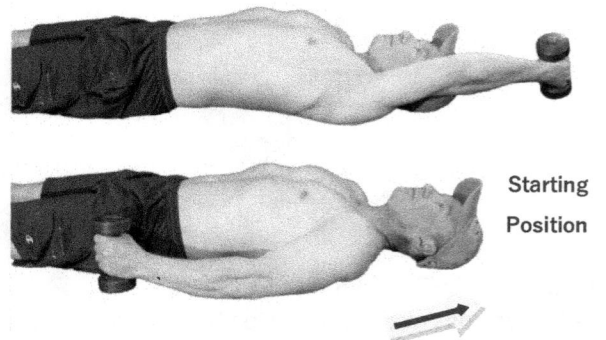

Starting Position

FLEXION – SUPINE – SINGLE OR BILATERAL - WEIGHT

Lie on your back with your arm at your side. Holding a weight, slowly raise arm up and forward towards overhead.

	_____ Reps _____ Sets _____X Day _____Hold		_____ Reps _____ Sets _____X Day _____Hold
37	**Notes:**	**38**	**Notes:**

Starting Position

FLEXION – SUPINE - DOWEL

Lie on your back holding dowel with both hands. Slowly raise up and forward towards overhead. Return to starting position. Repeat.
*If you have an injury/weakness, allow your unaffected arm to perform most of the effort. Your affected arm should be partially relaxed.

Starting Position

FLEXION – SUPINE - DOWEL – Add weight only if equal strength

Attach ankle weight to dowel. Lie on your back holding dowel with both hands. Slowly raise up and forward towards overhead. Return to starting position. Repeat.

	_____ Reps _____ Sets _____X Day _____Hold		_____ Reps _____ Sets _____X Day _____Hold
39	**Notes:**	**40**	**Notes:**

FLEXION - SELF FIXATION – ELASTIC BAND

Hold an elastic band in front and fixate unaffected arm straight by your side or on your leg. Pull the band upward towards the ceiling with your target arm.

Starting Position

FLEXION – ELASTIC BAND

In a standing position, step on the band with one leg. Keep your arm at your side holding an elastic band and draw up your arm up in front of you keeping your elbow straight.

	_____ Reps _____ Sets _____X Day _____Hold
41	**Notes:**

FLEXION - STANDING - PALMS DOWN / OVERHAND DOWEL - Add weight only if equal strength

Hold a dowel/cane with both arms, palm down on both sides. Raise the dowel forward and up. (see #39/40) *Do not use weight if you have an injury/weakness. Allow your unaffected arm to perform most of the work. Your affected arm should be partially relaxed.

	_____ Reps _____ Sets _____X Day _____Hold
42	**Notes:**

FLEXION - STANDING - PALMS UP /UNDERHAND DOWEL - Add weight only if equal strength

Hold a dowel/cane with both arms and palms up on both sides. Raise the dowel forward and up. *Do not use weight if you have an injury/weakness. Allow your unaffected arm to perform most of the work. Your affected arm should be partially relaxed.

	_____ Reps _____ Sets _____X Day _____Hold
43	**Notes:**

FLEXION – PALMS FACING INWARD - Can remove weight BILATERAL or ALTERNATE ARMS.

Sit or stand with your arm at your side. Hold a free weight with your palm facing your side and your elbows straight. Raise up your arm forward as shown then return to starting position. Do not let your shoulder shrug upwards unless instructed to go over shoulder level height.

	_____ Reps _____ Sets _____X Day _____Hold
44	**Notes:**

FLEXION – PALMS DOWN - Can remove weight BILATERAL or ALTERNATE ARMS.

Sit or stand with your arm at your side. Hold a weight with your palm facing down and your elbows straight. Raise up your arm forward as shown then return to starting position. Do not let your shoulder shrug upwards unless instructed to go over shoulder height.

V Raises

45	_____ Reps _____ Sets _____ X Day _____ Hold Notes:	46	_____ Reps _____ Sets _____ X Day _____ Hold Notes:

V RAISE

Start with your arms down by your side, palms facing inward, thumbs up and your elbows straight. Raise up your arms in the form of a V to shoulder height as shown keeping elbows straight then return to starting position.

Starting Position

V RAISE – WEIGHTS

Holding free weights, start with your arms down by your side, palms facing inward and your elbows straight. Raise up your arms in the form of a V to shoulder height keeping elbows straight – return.

Shoulder Press

47	_____ Reps _____ Sets _____ X Day _____ Hold Notes:	48	_____ Reps _____ Sets _____ X Day _____ Hold Notes:

Starting Position

MILITARY PRESS – DOWEL- Add weight only if equal strength

Hold a dowel or cane at chest height. Slowly push the wand upwards towards the ceiling until your elbows become fully straightened. Return to the original position.

Starting Position

MILITARY PRESS - FREE WEIGHTS

Hold free weights at 90-degree angle as shown above.
Slowly push your arms upwards towards the ceiling until your elbows become fully straightened. Return to the original position.

Shoulder Extension

_____ Reps _____ Sets _____ X Day _____ Hold	_____ Reps _____ Sets _____ X Day _____ Hold
49 Notes:	**50** Notes:

ISOMETRIC EXTENSION - Can use towel roll for comfort

Gently push your bent elbow back into a wall. Hold for 5-10 seconds. Relax and repeat.

PRONE EXTENSION - EXERCISE BALL – Can add weights.

Lie face down over an exercise ball with your elbows straight and along the side of your body. Slowly raise your arms upward along your side and then return to original position.

_____ Reps _____ Sets _____ X Day _____ Hold	_____ Reps _____ Sets _____ X Day _____ Hold
51 Notes:	**52** Notes:

SHOULDER EXTENSION - STANDING

Start with arms by your side. Draw your arm back behind your waist. Keep your elbows straight.

SHOULDER EXTENSION - STANDING - WEIGHTS

Hold a weight by your side and draw your arm back. Keep your elbows straight.

	_____ Reps _____ Sets _____ X Day _____ Hold
53	**Notes:**

Starting Position

EXTENSION – STANDING – DOWEL - Add weight only if equal strength

Hold a dowel or cane behind your back with both arms. Draw your arms back.

	_____ Reps _____ Sets _____ X Day _____ Hold
54	**Notes:**

EXTENSION - SELF FIXATION - ELASTIC BAND

Hold an elastic band out in front of you with your fixated arm.   Pull the band downward towards the ground and backwards with your target arm.

	_____ Reps _____ Sets _____ X Day _____ Hold
55	**Notes:**

EXTENSION - ELASTIC BAND

Fixate the end of an elastic band at top of door. Hold the elastic band in front of you with your elbows straight. Slowly pull the band down and back towards your side.

	_____ Reps _____ Sets _____ X Day _____ Hold
56	**Notes:**

EXTENSION - BILATERAL - ELASTIC BAND

Fixate the middle of an elastic band at top of door. Hold the elastic band with both arms in front of you with your elbows straight. Slowly pull the band downwards and back towards your side.

Shoulder Internal Rotation (IR)

57	_____ Reps _____ Sets _____ X Day _____ Hold	58	_____ Reps _____ Sets _____ X Day _____ Hold
	Notes:		Notes:

INTERNAL ROTATION – ISOMETRIC - Can use towel roll for comfort

Press your hand into a wall using the palm side of your hand and hold. Maintain a bent elbow the entire time.

INTERNAL ROTATION - ISOMETRIC- ELEVATED - Can use towel roll for comfort

Push the front of your hand into a wall with your elbow bent and arm elevated and hold.

59	_____ Reps _____ Sets _____ X Day _____ Hold	60	_____ Reps _____ Sets _____ X Day _____ Hold
	Notes:		Notes:

INTERNAL ROTATION - SIDELYING

Lie on your side with your shoulder flexed to 90 degrees and elbow bent and rested on the table/bed/matt. Your forearm should be pointing up towards the ceiling. Allow your forearm to lower toward the table as shown. Place a rolled-up towel under your elbow if needed.

INTERNAL ROTATION - ELASTIC BAND

Hold an elastic band at your side with your elbow bent. Start with your hand away from your stomach and then pull the band towards your stomach. Keep your elbow near your side the entire time.

61	_____ Reps _____ Sets _____X Day _____Hold
	Notes:

62	_____ Reps _____ Sets _____X Day _____Hold
	Notes:

INTERNAL / EXTERNAL ROTATION - STANDING – DOWEL
Add weight only if equal strength

Stand and hold a dowel/cane with both hands keeping your elbows bent. Move your arms and dowel/cane side-to-side. _If you have an injury/weakness, the affected arm should be partially relaxed while your unaffected arm performs most of the effort._

Starting Position

INTERNAL ROTATION – DOWEL - Add weight only if equal strength

While holding a dowel/cane behind your back, slowly pull the wand up.

Shoulder External Rotation (ER)

63	_____ Reps _____ Sets _____X Day _____Hold
	Notes:

64	_____ Reps _____ Sets _____X Day _____Hold
	Notes:

EXTERNAL ROTATION - ISOMETRIC – Can use towel roll for comfort

Gently press your hand into a wall using the back side of your hand. Maintain a bent elbow the entire time.

EXTERNAL ROTATION - ISOMETRIC – ELEVATED - Can use towel roll for comfort

Gently push the back of your hand/arm into a wall with your arm elevated.

	_____ Reps _____ Sets _____ X Day _____ Hold
65	**Notes:**

Starting Position

EXTERNAL ROTATION WITH TOWEL - SIDELYING

Lie on your side with your elbow bent to 90 degrees. Place a rolled-up towel between your arm and the side your body as shown. Squeeze your shoulder blade back and rotate arm up and hold this position. Slowly rotate back to original position and repeat.

	_____ Reps _____ Sets _____ X Day _____ Hold
66	**Notes:**

Starting Position

EXTERNAL ROTATION – 90/90 - WEIGHTS

Hold weights with elbows bent to 90 degrees and away from your side. Rotate your shoulders back so that the palms of your hands face forward and then return as shown.

	_____ Reps _____ Sets _____ X Day _____ Hold
67	**Notes:**

EXTERNAL ROTATION - BILATERAL - ELASTIC BAND
Can put a towel between side and elbow (see #68)

Hold an elastic band with your elbows bent, pull your hands away from your stomach area. Keep your elbows near the side of your body.

	_____ Reps _____ Sets _____ X Day _____ Hold
68	**Notes:**

EXTERNAL ROTATION - ELASTIC BAND – Can add roll between side and arm

Fixate an elastic band to the door at elbow height. Hold the other end of the band at your side with your elbow bent. Start with your hand near your stomach and then pull the band away. Keep your elbow at your side the entire time.

Shoulder Adduction (ADD)

	_____ Reps _____ Sets _____ X Day _____ Hold		_____ Reps _____ Sets _____ X Day _____ Hold
69	Notes:	**70**	Notes:

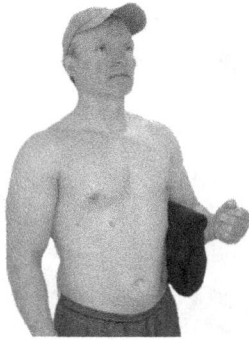

ADDUCTION – ISOMETRIC - Can use towel roll for comfort

Place a towel roll between your bent elbow and body. Gently push your elbow into the side of your body.

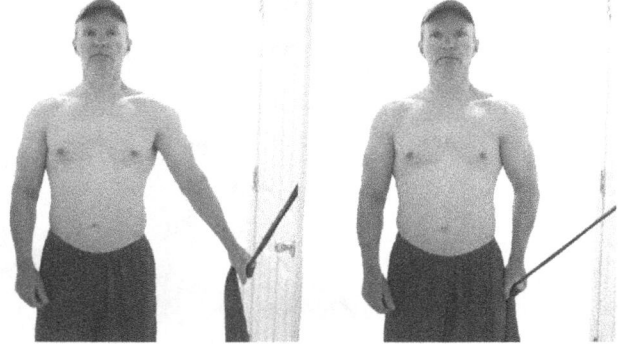

ADDUCTION - ELASTIC BAND

Fixate an elastic band to the door and hold the other end of the band away from your side. Pull the band towards your side keeping your elbow straight.

Shoulder Abduction (ABD)

	_____ Reps _____ Sets _____ X Day _____ Hold		_____ Reps _____ Sets _____ X Day _____ Hold
71	Notes:	**72**	Notes:

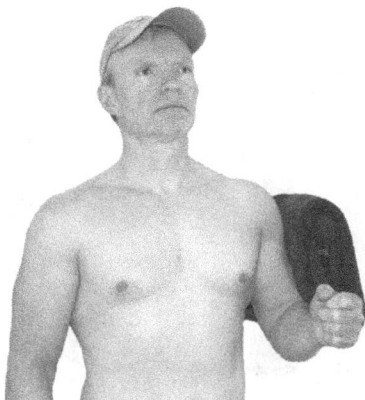

ABDUCTION – ISOMETRIC - Can use towel roll for comfort

Gently push your elbow out to the side into a wall with your elbow bent.

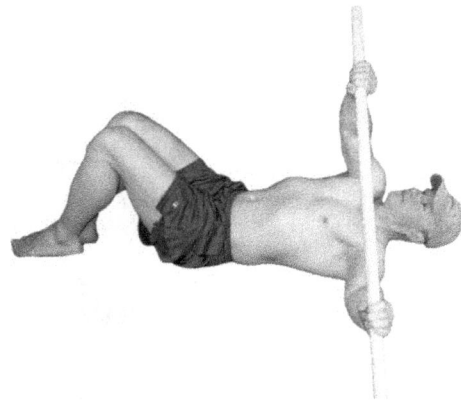

HORIZONTAL ABDUCTION - DOWEL

Lie on your back holding a dowel/cane straight up towards the ceiling with your elbows straight. Bring your arms and wand to the side and then towards the other.

	_____ Reps _____ Sets _____ X Day _____ Hold
73	Notes:

Starting Position

HORIZONTAL ABDUCTION/ADDUCTTION - SUPINE
Lie on your back with arm straight up in front of your body. Slowly lower your arm out towards the side. Return to original position.

	_____ Reps _____ Sets _____ X Day _____ Hold
74	Notes:

Starting Position

HORIZONTAL ABDUCTION/ADDUCTTION - SUPINE - WEIGHT

Hold a weight. Lie on your back with arm straight up in front of your body. Slowly lower your arm out towards the side. Return to original position

	_____ Reps _____ Sets _____ X Day _____ Hold
75	Notes:

Starting Position

ABDUCTION - SIDELYING - Can add weight

Lie on your side with arm at your side. Slowly raise the target arm up towards head and away from your side.

	_____ Reps _____ Sets _____ X Day _____ Hold
76	Notes:

Starting Position

HORIZONTAL ABDUCTION - SIDELYING - Can add weight

Lie on your side with arm out in front of your body. Slowly raise up the arm overhead towards the ceiling.

	_____ Reps _____ Sets _____ X Day _____ Hold
77	**Notes:**

ABDUCTION – WEIGHT – Can do without a weight

Hold a weight with your affected arm at your side.
Keeping your elbow straight, raise up your arm to the side.

	_____ Reps _____ Sets _____ X Day _____ Hold
78	**Notes:**

ABDUCTION – ELASTIC BAND

Fixate an elastic band under a door and hold band with hand farthest away from door at your side. Keeping your elbow straight, raise up your arm to the side.

	_____ Reps _____ Sets _____ X Day _____ Hold
79	**Notes:**

HORIZONTAL ABDUCTION – BILATERAL - ELASTIC BAND

Hold an elastic band in both hands with your elbows straight in front of your body. Slowly pull your arms apart towards the sides.

	_____ Reps _____ Sets _____ X Day _____ Hold
80	**Notes:**

90/90 ABDUCTION - WEIGHT

Hold weights at your side with elbows bent to 90 degrees. Raise up your elbows away from your side while maintaining your elbows bent at 90 degrees.

Lateral/Frontal Raise

_____ Reps _____ Sets _____X Day _____Hold		

81 Notes:

Starting Position

LATERAL RAISES

Hold weights at your side with arms straight. Raise up your elbows away from your side while keeping your elbow straight the entire time.

_____ Reps _____ Sets _____X Day _____Hold		

82 Notes:

Starting Position

LATERAL RAISES – LEAN FORWARD

Bend slightly at the waist holding weights slightly in front. Raise up your elbows away from your side squeezing shoulder blades together.

_____ Reps _____ Sets _____X Day _____Hold		

83 Notes:

Starting Position

LATERAL RAISES – LEAN FORWARD - ARM ROTATION

Bend slightly at the waist holding weights slightly in front as shown palms facing your body. Raise up your elbows away from your side squeezing shoulder blades together.

_____ Reps _____ Sets _____X Day _____Hold		

84 Notes:

FRONTAL RAISE – WEIGHTS – Can do without weights

Hold weights at your side with arms straight. Slowly raise your arms in front of of your body.

Upright Rows

	_____ Reps _____ Sets _____X Day _____Hold		_____ Reps _____ Sets _____X Day _____Hold
85	Notes:	86	Notes:

Starting
Position

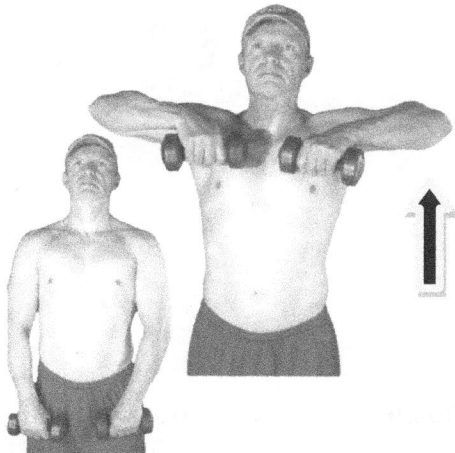

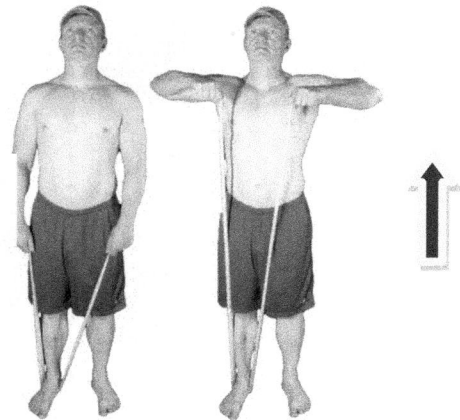

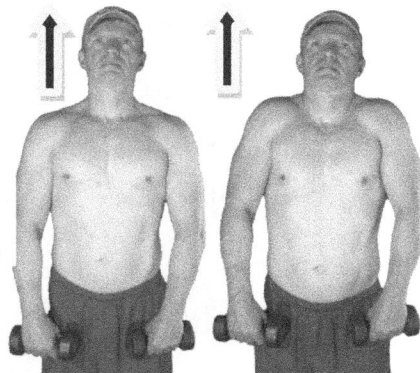

Starting
Position

UPRIGHT ROW – WEIGHTS - Can use kettle bell

Hold weights or kettlebell with both hands at waist height. Lift the weights to chest height as you bend at your elbows.

UPRIGHT ROW – ELASTIC BAND

Stand on an elastic band with either one or both feet. Hold band at waist height and raise it up to chest height as you bend at your elbows.

Shoulder Shrugs & Rolls

	_____ Reps _____ Sets _____X Day _____Hold		_____ Reps _____ Sets _____X Day _____Hold
87	Notes:	88	Notes:

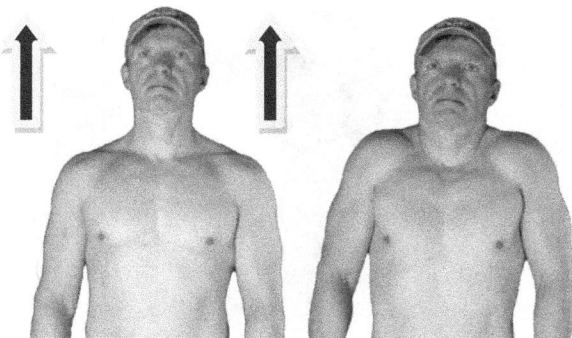

SHRUGS

Raise your shoulders upward towards your ears as shown. Shrug both shoulders at the same time.

Starting
Position

SHRUGS - WEIGHTS

Hold weights in both hands with arms straight. Raise your shoulders upward towards your ears. Shrug both shoulders at the same time.

	_____ Reps _____ Sets _____X Day _____Hold		_____ Reps _____ Sets _____X Day _____Hold
89	Notes:	**90**	Notes:

SHOULDER ROLLS

Move your shoulders in a circular pattern so that your are moving in an up, back and down direction. Perform small circles if needed for comfort.
Complete one set and then reverse direction

SHOULDER ROLLS - WEIGHTS

Hold weights in both or one hand. Move your shoulders in a circular pattern so that your are moving in an up, back and down direction.
Complete one set and then reverse direction

Scapular Retraction

	_____ Reps _____ Sets _____X Day _____Hold		_____ Reps _____ Sets _____X Day _____Hold
91	Notes:	**92**	Notes:

SCAPULAR RETRACTIONS - BILATERAL

Draw your shoulder blades back and down.

SCAPULAR RETRACTION – SINGLE ARM

With your arm raised up and elbow bent, draw your shoulder blade back and down.

	_____ Reps _____ Sets _____X Day _____Hold
93	**Notes:**

ELASTIC BAND SCAPULAR RETRACTIONS WITH MINI SHOULDER EXTENSIONS

Fixate an elastic band to the door and hold with both arms in front of you with your elbows straight. Slowly squeeze your shoulder blades together as you pull the band back. Be sure your shoulders do not rise up.

	_____ Reps _____ Sets _____X Day _____Hold
94	**Notes:**

PRONE RETRACTION – Can do without weight

Lie face down with your elbows straight. Slowly draw your shoulder blade back towards your spine. Your whole arm should rise including your shoulder blade upward as shown. Your elbow should be straight the entire time.

Scapular Protraction

	_____ Reps _____ Sets _____X Day _____Hold
95	**Notes:**

SCAPULAR PROTRACTION - SUPINE - BILATERAL

Lie on your back with your arms extended out in front of your body and towards the ceiling. While keeping your elbows straight, protract your shoulders reaching forward towards the ceiling. Keep your elbows straight the entire time.

	_____ Reps _____ Sets _____X Day _____Hold
96	**Notes:**

SCAPULAR PROTRACTION - SUPINE - WEIGHT

Lie on your back holding a weight with your arm extended out in front of your body and towards the ceiling. While keeping your elbows straight, protract your shoulders reaching forward towards the ceiling. Keep your elbows straight the entire time.

	_____ Reps _____ Sets _____X Day _____Hold
97	Notes:

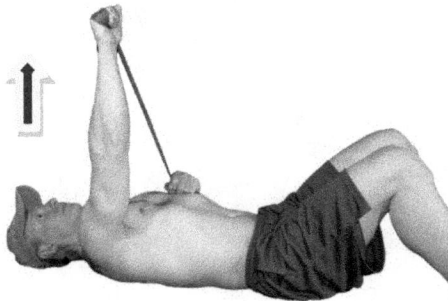

SCAPULAR PROTRACTION - SUPINE - ELASTIC BAND

Lie on your back and hold elastic band in both hands. Bend the unaffected arm to fixate the band. Extend the target arm out in front of your body and straight up towards the ceiling. While keeping your elbows straight, protract your shoulder blade forward towards the ceiling. Keep your elbows straight the entire time.

	_____ Reps _____ Sets _____X Day _____Hold
98	Notes:

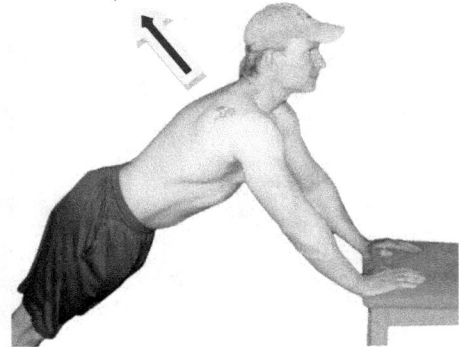

SCAPULAR PROTRACTION / TABLE PLANK

Start in a push up position on your hands and leaning up against a table or countertop as shown. Maintain this position as you protract your shoulder blades forward to raise your body upward a few inches. Return to original position.
*Progress by standing further away from the table.

Chest Press

	_____ Reps _____ Sets _____X Day _____Hold
99	Notes:

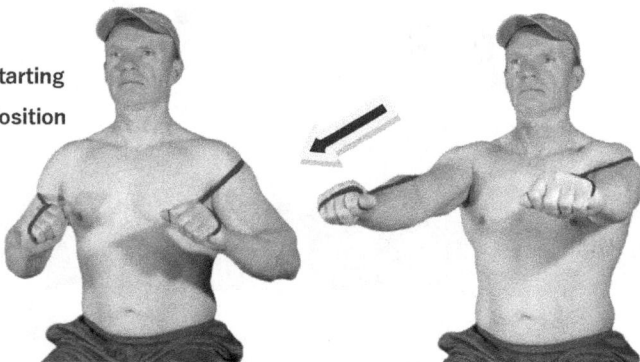

CHEST PRESS – SEATED or STANDING - ELASTIC BAND

Hold elastic band with both hands at your side and elbows bent with band wrapped around body or chair. Push the band out in front of your body as you straighten your elbows.

	_____ Reps _____ Sets _____X Day _____Hold
100	Notes:

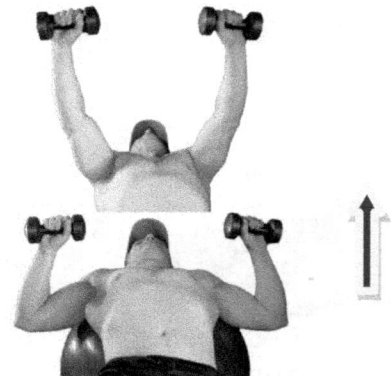

CHEST PRESS – BALL, FLOOR or BENCH- WEIGHTS

Lie on your back with your elbows bent. Slowly raise up your arms towards the ceiling while extending your elbows straight up above your head.

_____ Reps _____ Sets _____ X Day _____ Hold

101 | Notes:

_____ Reps _____ Sets _____ X Day _____ Hold

102 | Notes:

Starting

Position

DOWEL PRESS – STANDING – Add weight only if equal strength

Hold a dowel/cane at chest height. Slowly push the dowel outwards in front of your body so that your elbows become fully straightened. Return to the original position.

Starting

Position

CHEST PRESS – STANDING or SEATED

Hold weights in both hands with your arms at your side and elbows bent. Push your arms out in front of your body as you straighten your elbows.

Rows

_____ Reps _____ Sets _____ X Day _____ Hold

103 | Notes:

_____ Reps _____ Sets _____ X Day _____ Hold

104 | Notes:

BENT OVER ROWS

Stand, bend over and support yourself with the unaffected arm. Slowly draw up your target arm as you bend your elbow. Keep your back flat the entire time.

ROWS – PRONE – On bed or table

Lie face down with your elbows straight, slowly raise your arms upward while bending your elbows.

	_____ Reps _____ Sets _____ X Day _____ Hold
105	Notes:

ROWS - ELASTIC BAND

Fixate the elastic band in the door at elbow level. Hold the elastic band with both hands, draw back the band as you bend your elbows. Keep your elbows near the side of your body.

	_____ Reps _____ Sets _____ X Day _____ Hold
106	Notes:

WIDE ROWS - ELASTIC BAND

Fixate the elastic band in the door and hold the band with both hands. Draw back the band as you bend your elbows squeezing shoulder blades together. Keep your arms about 90 degrees away from the side of your body.

	_____ Reps _____ Sets _____ X Day _____ Hold
107	Notes:

LOW ROW – ELASTIC BAND

Fixate the elastic band in the door below elbow level. Hold the elastic band with both hands, draw back the band as you bend your elbows. Keep your elbows near the side of your body.

	_____ Reps _____ Sets _____ X Day _____ Hold
108	Notes:

HIGH ROW – ELASTIC BAND

Fixate the elastic band at the top of the door. Hold the elastic band with both hands, draw back the band as you bend your elbows. Keep your elbows near the side of your body.

Flys

	_____ Reps _____ Sets _____X Day _____Hold			_____ Reps _____ Sets _____X Day _____Hold
109	**Notes:**		**110**	**Notes:**

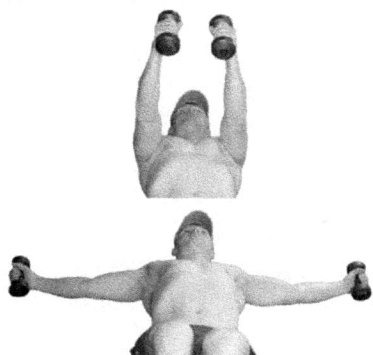

Starting

Position

FLY'S – FLOOR - WEIGHT

Holding weights, lie on your back with your arms horizontally out to the side. Bring your arms up and forward towards the ceiling. Lower your arms back down to the original position. Your elbows should be partially bent the entire time.

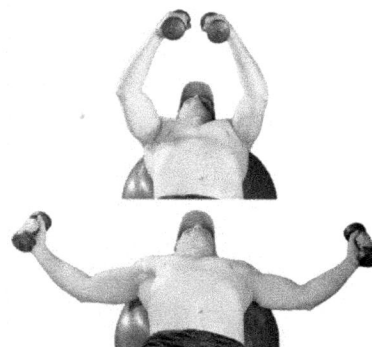

FLY'S – BALL or BENCH – WEIGHT

Holding weights, lie on your back on a ball with your arms horizontally out to the side. Bring your arms up and forward towards the ceiling. Lower your arms back down to the original position with elbows partially bent the entire time.

Wall pushups – To progress, move feet further away from wall

	_____ Reps _____ Sets _____X Day _____Hold			_____ Reps _____ Sets _____X Day _____Hold
111	**Notes:**		**112**	**Notes:**

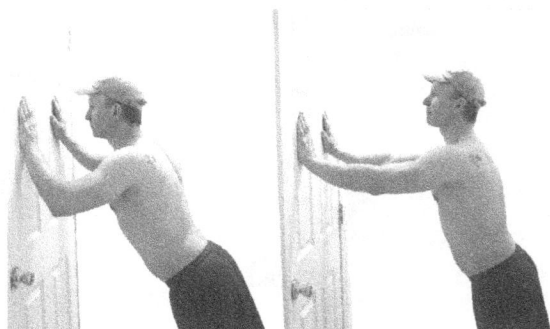

WALL PUSH UPS

Place your arms out in front of you with your elbows straight so that your hands just reach the wall. Bend your elbows slowly to bring your chest closer to the wall. Straighten your arms pushing your body away from wall. Maintain your feet planted on the ground the entire time.

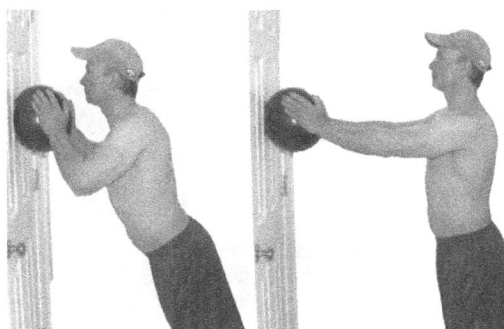

WALL PUSH UP - BALL

Place a ball on a wall while holding the ball with both hands as shown. Bend your elbows slowly to bring your chest closer to the wall and then straighten your arms pushing your body away from wall. Maintain your feet planted on the ground the entire time.

	_____ Reps _____ Sets _____X Day _____Hold
113	Notes:

WALL PUSH UP - Triceps uneven

Place your arms out in front of you with your elbows straight in an uneven position so that your hands just reach the wall. Bend your elbows slowly to bring your chest closer to the wall and then straighten your arms pushing your body away from wall. Maintain your feet planted on the ground the entire time.

	_____ Reps _____ Sets _____X Day _____Hold
114	Notes:

WALL PUSH UP – Hands inverted

Place your arms out in front of you with your elbows straight and hands inverted just reaching the wall. Bend your elbows slowly to bring your chest closer to the wall and then straighten your arms pushing your body away from wall. Maintain your feet planted on the ground the entire time.

	_____ Reps _____ Sets _____X Day _____Hold
115	Notes:

WALL PUSH UP - Narrow

Place your arms out in front of you with your elbows straight and hands close togther just reaching the wall. Bend your elbows slowly to bring your chest closer to the wall and then straighten your arms pushing your body away from wall. Maintain your feet planted on the ground the entire time.

	_____ Reps _____ Sets _____X Day _____Hold
116	Notes:

WALL PUSH UP – Wide

Place your arms out in front of you with your elbows straight and your arms and hands far apart just reaching the wall. Bend your elbows slowly to bring your chest closer to the wall and then straighten your arms pushing your body away from wall. Maintain your feet planted on the ground the entire time.

	Push ups	

	_____ Reps _____ Sets _____X Day _____Hold		_____ Reps _____ Sets _____X Day _____Hold
117	Notes:	**118**	Notes:

PUSH UPS - BALL

Start in a kneeling position with an exercise ball in front of you. Slowly walk yourself out with your arms so that the ball is positioned under your legs. Then perform push ups. *Progress by moving ball back towards thighs

Starting Position

PUSH UP - MODIFIED

Lie face down and use your arms and push yourself up. Keep your knees in contact with the floor and maintain a straight back the entire time.

	_____ Reps _____ Sets _____X Day _____Hold		_____ Reps _____ Sets _____X Day _____Hold
119	Notes:	**120**	Notes:

Starting Position

PUSH UP

Lie face down, use your arms and push yourself. Keep your toes in contact with the floor and maintain a straight back the entire time.

PUSH UP -DIAMOND

Lie face down and place your hands on the floor in the shape of a diamond with your thumbs and index fingers.
Use your arms and push yourself up.. Keep your toes in contact with the floor and maintain a straight back the entire time.

_____ Reps _____ Sets _____X Day _____Hold

121 Notes:

PUSH UP – MODIFIED - BOSU - UNSTABLE

Perform push-ups with your hands on a Bosu. Keep your knees in contact with the floor and maintain a straight back the entire time.

_____ Reps _____ Sets _____X Day _____Hold

122 Notes:

PUSH UP – BOSU - UNSTABLE

Perform push-ups with your hands on top of a Bosu. Keep your toes in contact with the floor and maintain a straight back the entire time.

_____ Reps _____ Sets _____X Day _____Hold

123 Notes:

PUSH UP – MODIFIED – INVERTED BOSU - UNSTABLE

Perform push-ups while holding an inverted Bosu. Try and maintain the Bosu platform as level as you can. Keep your knees in contact with the floor and maintain a straight back the entire time.

_____ Reps _____ Sets _____X Day _____Hold

124 Notes:

PUSH UP – INVERTED BOSU - UNSTABLE

Perform push-ups while holding an inverted Bosu. Try and maintain the Bosu platform as level as you can. Keep your toes in contact with the floor and maintain a straight back the entire time.

BALANCE – CORE – STANDING LE STRENGTH

Basics
- Requires LE strengthening for progression
- Perform exercises 2-3x a week
- Should be performed at beginning of exercise routine or can be the main exercise routine for endurance with increased repetitions or strength with resistance.

Duration, Frequency, Intensity, Sets and Reps
- Balance – 1 set, 2-4 repetitions for hold of 5-60 seconds
- Endurance – Less than 30 second rests in between sets
  - Static - 1 set, 5-10 repetitions as tolerated
  - Dynamic – 1 set, 3-10 reps for 10-30+ second hold as tolerated
- Strengthening – Add resistance with bands or weights (*see Strengthening for more information*)
  - Static – 2-3 sets, 3-12 reps – slow controlled movements
  - Dynamic – 1-3 sets, 2-4 reps

Static Balance Progression:
1. Bilateral – Both feet on the ground
2. Unilateral – One foot on the ground
3. Arm Movement – Overhead, can do arm exercises (*See Arm Strengthening for exercises*)
4. Trunk rotation – Rotate with or without arm movement
5. Eyes Shut (lack of visual cues – sensory removal)
6. Head Turns, hand/eye tracking, shifting focal point (vestibular – sensory alteration)
7. Reading (coordination)
8. Unstable – progression
   Repeat above on unstable surface such as balance pad, pillow, balance disc or Bosu.

Decrease Base of Support (BOS) Progression:
- Wide BOS
- Narrow Bos
- Staggered/Split Stance/Semi-tandem
- Tandem Stance
- Single Leg Stance

SOLID GROUND:
1. Support: Hold onto chair, counter, sink or another stationary object.
2. No Support: Stand next to stable surface if needed for security.
   - Can start with 1-2 hands and as you become more stable, decrease the number of fingers used for support. For example, take away the thumb and hold with 4 fingers, 3 fingers, 2 fingers, 1 finger and then without support.
3. Resistance: Add ankle weights on use elastic band for resistance

UNSTABLE SURFACE: Balance pad, Bosu, Half foam roll, Pillow or Other unstable surface
1. Support: Hold onto chair, counter or another stationary object.
2. No Support: Stand next to stable surface if needed for security.
   - Can start with 1-2 hands and as you become more stable, decrease the number of fingers used for support. For example, take away the thumb and hold with 4 fingers, 3 fingers, 2 fingers, 1 finger and then without support.
3. Resistance: Add ankle weights on use elastic band for resistance

Peripheral Neuropathy **Caution Balancing on Uneven Surface**	• Peripheral neuropathy can be a side effect of diabetes or may be as a result of damage to the peripheral nerves. These nerves carry information from the brain to other parts of the body. • Feet or lower extremity – Caution standing on uneven surface, such as a Bosu ball or balance pads due to decreased sensation in feet. Increased risk of falling. • Hands – Caution with holding dumbbells or grasping resistance bands.

Balance

EXERCISE Balance	EXERCISE NUMBER	NOTES
WIDE BOS DECREASING TO NARROW BOS	1	
NARROW BOS	2	
ARM MOVEMENT	3	
TRUNK ROTATION	4	
EYES SHUTS	5	
HEAD TURNS	6	
READING ALOUD	7	
BALANCE PAD	8	
SPLIT STANCE – SEMI TANDEM	9	
SPLIT STANCE - *Progression*	10	
TANDEM- SHARPENED ROMBERG STANCE	11	
TANDEM STANCE - Progression	12	
SINGLE LEG STANCE (SLS)	13	
SINGLE LEG STANCE (SLS) - *Progression*	14	
SLS – LEG FORWARD	15	
SLS – LEG BACKWARDS	16	
SLS – LEG FORWARD / OPPOSITE ARM UP	17	
SLS – LEG BACKWARDS / OPPOSITE ARM UP	18	
SLS - REACH FORWARD	19	
SLS - REACH TWIST	20	
SINGLE LEG TOE TAP	21	
SINGLE LEG STANCE - CLOCKS	22	
BALL ROLLS - HEEL TOE	23	
BALL ROLLS - LATERAL	24	
SQUAT	25	
SIT TO STAND	26	

Balance

EXERCISE Balance	EXERCISE NUMBER	NOTES
SQUATS – WALL WITH BALL	27	
SQUATS WITH WEIGHTS	28	
MINI SQUAT - UNSTABLE SUPPORT - FOAM PAD	29	
SQUATS - SINGLE LEG	30	
SIDE TO SIDE WEIGHT SHIFT	31	
FORWARD AND BACKWARDS WEIGHT SHIFTS	32	
SPLIT STANCE WEIGHT SHIFT SIDE TO SIDE	33	
SPLIT STANCE WEIGHT SHIFT FORWARD AND BACKWARDS	34	
WALL FALLS - FORWARD - BALANCE DRILL	35	
WALL FALLS - LATERAL - BALANCE DRILL	36	
WALL FALLS - BACKWARDS - BALANCE DRILL	37	
WALL FALLS - SINGLE LEG - FORWARD - BALANCE DRILL	38	
WALL FALLS - SINGLE LEG - LATERAL - BALANCE DRILL	39	
WALL FALLS - SINGLE LEG - MEDIAL - BALANCE DRILL	40	
WALL FALLS - SINGLE LEG - BACKWARDS - BALANCE DRILL	41	
FALL LATERAL - STEP RECOVERY	42	
FALL FORWARD - STEP RECOVERY	43	
FALL BACKWARD - STEP RECOVERY	44	
TOE TAP ABDUCTION	45	
HIP ABDUCTION - STANDING	46	
HIP EXTENSION – STANDING	47	
HIP FLEXION - STANDING – STRAIGHT LEG RAISE	48	
HIP / KNEE FLEXION - SINGLE LEG	49	
STANDING MARCHING	50	

EXERCISE Balance	EXERCISE NUMBER	NOTES
HAMSTRING CURL	51	
TOE RAISES	52	
TOE RAISES IR AND ER	53	
ONE LEGGED TOE RAISE	54	
SINGLE LEG BALANCE FORWARD	55	
SINGLE LEG BALANCE LATERAL	56	
SINGLE LEG BALANCE RETRO	57	
SINGLE LEG STANCE RETROLATERAL	58	
SQUAT	59	
SINGLE LEG SQUAT	60	
LUNGE – STATIC	61	
LUNGE FORWARD/BACKWARD	62	
FOUR CORNER MARCHING IN PLACE	63	
FOUR CORNER MARCHING IN PLACE WITH HEAD TURNS	64	
WALKING ON HEELS FORWARD AND BACKWARDS	65	
WALKING ON TOES FORWARD AND BACKWARDS	66	
TANDEM STANCE AND WALK – FORWARD AND BACKWARDS	67	
RUNNING MAN	68	
HOP STICK - FORWARD	69	
HOP STICK - BACKWARDS	70	
MINI LATERAL LUNGE	71	
SIDE STEPPING	72	
HOP STICK - LATERAL	73	
SINGLE LEG DEAD LIFT	74	

Balance

EXERCISE	EXERCISE NUMBER	NOTES
Balance		
CONE TAPS - SINGLE LEG STANCE	75	
CONE TAPS - SINGLE LEG STANCE - UNSTABLE	76	
FIGURE 8 AROUND CONES	77	
FIGURE 8 AROUND CONES – FOOT OR HAND TAP	78	
BALANCE DOUBLE LEG STANCE - WIDE	79	
BALANCE DOUBLE LEG STANCE - NARROW	80	
TANDEM STANCE	81	
TANDEM WALK	82	
SINGLE LEG STANCE - ABDUCTION	83	
SINGLE LEG STANCE - ABDUCTION	84	
SINGLE LEG STANCE – FORWARD KICK	85	
SINGLE LEG STANCE – HAMSTRING CURL	86	
SINGLE LEG SQUAT – LEG FORWARD	87	
SINGLE LEG SQUAT – LEG BACKWARDS	88	
TOE TAP OR HEEL PLACEMENT	89	
PULL UP FOOT TOUCHES ON STEP	90	
ALTERNATING SUSTAINED FOOT TOUCHES ON STEP	91	
STEP UP AND OVER	92	
FORWARD SWING THROUGH STEP	93	
SIDE STEPPING - *REPEAT STEPS 89-93 from a side approach.*	94	

BALANCE PROGRESSION- STATIC – See WARNING above Re: Peripheral Neuropathy

Hip Width/Narrow Stance >>>>> Staggered Stance >>>>> Tandem Stance >>>>> Single-Leg Stance

1. Hold onto a chair, counter or other steady object.
2. Continue steps 2-8 holding on to a sturdy object.
3. Can start with 1-2 hands and as you become more stable, decrease the number of fingers used for support. For example, take away the thumb and hold with 4 fingers, 3 fingers, 2 fingers, 1 finger and then without support.
4. When feeling comfortable, take away support staying close to object for security
5. When able to complete with decreased support, add balance pad or unstable surface completing 2-8 as above.

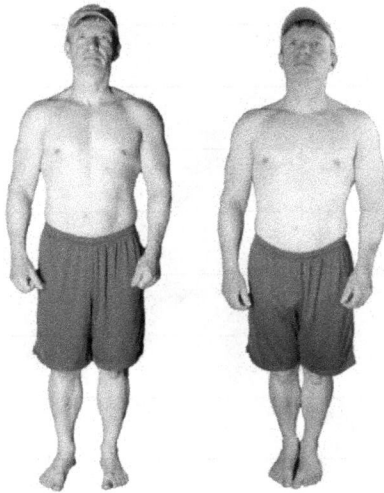

HIP WIDTH OR WIDE BASE OF SUPPORT (BOS) > NARROW BASE OF SUPPORT (BOS)

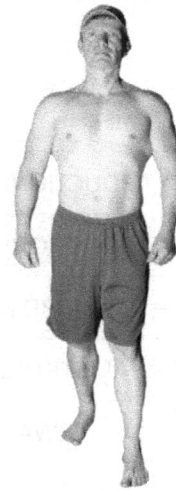

STAGGERED STANCE – SPLIT STANCE

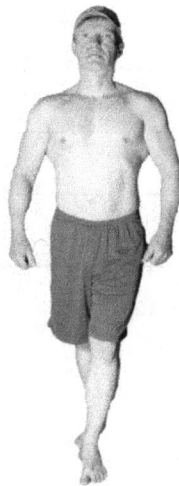

TANDEM STANCE

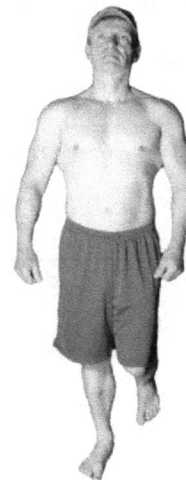

SINGLE LEG STANCE

Balance

	_____ Reps _____ Sets _____ X Day _____ Hold		_____ Reps _____ Sets _____ X Day _____ Hold
1	**Notes:**	2	**Notes:**

WIDE BOS DECREASING TO NARROW BOS

Continue steps 2-8 holding on to a sturdy object and then progress with decreased support as outlined above.

NARROW BOS

Stand with your feet together Count to 10. Increase time up to 60 seconds as tolerated maintaining your balance in this position.

	_____ Reps _____ Sets _____ X Day _____ Hold		_____ Reps _____ Sets _____ X Day _____ Hold
3	**Notes:**	4	**Notes:**

ARM MOVEMENT

Examples:
- Throw ball up in arm and catch
- Play catch with partner
- Reach hands above head and then down by side
- Do standing arm exercises (*See Arm Strengthening for examples*)

TRUNK ROTATION – reach side to side

Examples:
- Reach side to side within BOS
- Reach side to side and forward out of BOS

	_____ Reps _____ Sets _____X Day _____Hold		_____ Reps _____ Sets _____X Day _____Hold
5	Notes:	**6**	Notes:

EYES SHUTS - Lack of visual cues – *Sensory Removal*

Stand with eyes shut and count to 10. Increase time up to 60 seconds as tolerated.

HEAD TURNS - Vestibular – *Sensory Alteration*

Examples:
- Turn head slowly from side to side
- Move head up and down slowly
- Put one finger out in front of face at arm's length moving in outward/inward direction and move head to follow with eyes. Slow hand tracking.
- Shift focal point to different objects in the room
- *Can add head turns with eyes closed*

	_____ Reps _____ Sets _____X Day _____Hold		_____ Reps _____ Sets _____X Day _____Hold
7	Notes:	**8**	Notes:

READING ALOUD - *Coordination / Cognitive Task*

Hold reading material, such as a book, paper, tablet, or magazine in one or both hands. Read out loud and progress to moving your head and the object on occasion to the side or up/down.

BALANCE PAD or another unstable surface

Place balance pad, Bosu, pillow or other unstable surface by a chair or counter for support. Stand on the pad.

****REPEAT STEPS 2-8 on unstable surface****

Balance

	_____ Reps _____ Sets _____ X Day _____ Hold		_____ Reps _____ Sets _____ X Day _____ Hold
9	**Notes:**	10	**Notes:**

SPLIT STANCE – SEMI TANDEM

Place one foot forward and the opposite foot to the back and slightly out to the side. Count to 10. Increase time up to 60 seconds as tolerated maintaining your balance in this position.

SPLIT STANCE

FOLLOW STEPS 2-8 AS SEEN WITH NARROW BOS AS OUTLINED IN BALANCE PROGRESSION

1. HOLD STEADY OBJECT PROGRESSING TO NO SUPPORT
2. STAND FOR 10-60 SECONDS
3. ARM MOVEMENT
4. TRUNK ROTATION
5. EYES SHUT
6. HEAD TURNS
7. READING
8. **UNSTABLE**

REPEAT ABOVE ON UNSTABLE SURFACE SUCH AS BALANCE PAD, PILLOW, BALANCE DISC, HALF FOARM ROLL OR BOSU.

	_____ Reps _____ Sets _____ X Day _____ Hold		_____ Reps _____ Sets _____ X Day _____ Hold
11	**Notes:**	12	**Notes:**

TANDEM- SHARPENED ROMBERG STANCE

Place the heel of one foot so that it touches the toes of the other foot. Count to 10. Increase time up to 60 seconds as tolerated maintaining your balance in this position.

TANDEM STANCE

FOLLOW STEPS 2-8 AS SEEN WITH NARROW BOS AS OUTLINED IN BALANCE PROGRESSION

1. HOLD STEADY OBJECT PROGRESSING TO NO SUPPORT
2. STAND FOR 10-60 SECONDS
3. ARM MOVEMENT
4. TRUNK ROTATION
5. EYES SHUT
6. HEAD TURNS
7. READING
8. **UNSTABLE**

REPEAT ABOVE ON UNSTABLE SURFACE SUCH AS BALANCE PAD, PILLOW, BALANCE DISC, HALF FOARM ROLL OR BOSU.

	_____ Reps _____ Sets _____X Day _____Hold		_____ Reps _____ Sets _____X Day _____Hold
13	Notes:	**14**	Notes:

SINGLE LEG STANCE (SLS)

Stand on one foot. Count to 10 > 60 seconds as tolerated maintaining your balance in this position. Maintain a slightly bent knee on the stance side.

SINGLE LEG STANCE

FOLLOW STEPS 2-8 AS SEEN WITH NARROW BOS AS OUTLINED IN BALANCE PROGRESSION

1. HOLD STEADY OBJECT PROGRESSING TO NO SUPPORT
2. STAND FOR 10-60 SECONDS
3. ARM MOVEMENT
4. TRUNK ROTATION
5. EYES SHUT
6. HEAD TURNS
7. READING
8. **UNSTABLE**

REPEAT ABOVE ON UNSTABLE SURFACE SUCH AS BALANCE PAD, PILLOW, BALANCE DISC, HALF FOARM ROLL OR BOSU.

Single Leg Stance (SLS) with Arm and/or Leg Movements- *Progress to Balance Pad*

	_____ Reps _____ Sets _____X Day _____Hold		_____ Reps _____ Sets _____X Day _____Hold
15	Notes:	**16**	Notes:

SLS – LEG FORWARD

Stand on one leg and maintain your balance. Hold your leg out in front of your body and then return to the original position. Repeat on opposite side. Maintain a slightly bent knee on the stance side.

SLS – LEG BACKWARDS

Stand on one leg and maintain your balance. Hold your leg in the back of your body and then return to original position. Repeat on opposite side. Maintain a slightly bent knee on the stance side.

	_____ Reps _____ Sets _____X Day _____Hold		_____ Reps _____ Sets _____X Day _____Hold
17	**Notes:**	**18**	**Notes:**

SLS – LEG FORWARD / OPPOSITE ARM UP

Stand on one leg and maintain your balance. Hold your leg out in front of your body and opposite arm up over your head. Return to the original position. Repeat on opposite side. Maintain a slightly bent knee on the stance side.

SLS – LEG BACKWARDS / OPPOSITE ARM UP

Stand on one leg and maintain your balance. Hold your leg out in front of your body and opposite arm up over your head. Return to the original position. Repeat on opposite side. Maintain a slightly bent knee on the stance side.

	_____ Reps _____ Sets _____X Day _____Hold		_____ Reps _____ Sets _____X Day _____Hold
19	**Notes:**	**20**	**Notes:**

SLS - REACH FORWARD

Stand on one leg and maintain your balance. Reach forward with your opposite arm as far as you can without losing your balance and then return to original position. Repeat on opposite side. Maintain a slightly bent knee on the stance side.

SLS - REACH TWIST

Stand on one leg and maintain your balance. Reach forward and across your body with your opposite arm as far as you can without losing your balance and then return to original position. Repeat on opposite side. Maintain a slightly bent knee on the stance side.

	_____ Reps _____ Sets _____X Day _____Hold
21	Notes:

SINGLE LEG TOE TAP

Start by standing on one leg and maintain your balance. Tap the opposite foot on a slightly raised object, such as a box or balance pad. To progress, increase the height of object, such as a stair step or cone. Can alternate feet or repeat on same side for several repetitions and then repeat on opposite side.

	_____ Reps _____ Sets _____X Day _____Hold
22	Notes:

SINGLE LEG STANCE - CLOCKS

Start by standing on one leg and maintain your balance. Image a clock on the floor where your stance leg is in the center. Lightly touch position 1 as illustrated with the opposite foot. Then return that leg to the starting position. Next, touch position 2 and return. Maintain a slightly bent knee on the stance side.

	_____ Reps _____ Sets _____X Day _____Hold
23	Notes:

BALL ROLLS - HEEL TOE

In a standing position, place one foot on a ball and roll it forward and back in a controlled motion from heel to toe while maintaining your balance.

	_____ Reps _____ Sets _____X Day _____Hold
24	Notes:

BALL ROLLS - LATERAL

In a standing position, place one foot on a ball and roll it side to side in a controlled motion from the inner side of your foot to the outer side of your foot while maintaining your balance.

Squats

_____ Reps _____ Sets _____X Day _____Hold	_____ Reps _____ Sets _____X Day _____Hold
25 **Notes:**	**26** **Notes:**

SQUAT – Can use chair or counter for support and chair behind if needed.

Stand with feet shoulder width apart (in front of a stable support for balance if needed.) Bend your knees and lower your body towards the floor. Your body weight should mostly be directed through the heels of your feet. Return to a standing position. Knees should bend in line with toes and not pass the front of the foot.

SIT TO STAND - Can use armchair to push off if needed

Start by scooting close to the front of the chair. Lean forward at your trunk and reach forward with your arms and rise to standing. (You may use a chair with arms to push off if needed and progress as tolerated).

Use your arms as a counterbalance by reaching forward when in sitting and lower them as you approach standing.

_____ Reps _____ Sets _____X Day _____Hold	_____ Reps _____ Sets _____X Day _____Hold
27 **Notes:**	**28** **Notes:**

SQUATS – **WALL WITH BALL**

Place either a small ball or therapy ball between you and the wall. Bend your knees and lower your body towards the floor. Return to a standing position. Knees should bend in line with toes and not pass the front of the foot.

SQUATS WITH WEIGHTS

Hold dumbbells or other weights in both hands by your side. Bend your knees and lower your body towards the floor. Return to a standing position. Knees should bend in line with toes and not pass the front of the foot

	_____ Reps _____ Sets _____X Day _____Hold
29	**Notes:**

MINI SQUAT - UNSTABLE SUPPORT - FOAM PAD

Start with your feet shoulder-width apart, toes pointed straight ahead and standing on a balance pad. Next, bend your knees to approximately 30 degrees of flexion to perform a mini squat as shown. Then, return to original position. Knees should not pass the front of the foot.

	_____ Reps _____ Sets _____X Day _____Hold
30	**Notes:**

SQUATS - SINGLE LEG

While standing on one leg in front of a stable support for assisted balance, bend your knee and lower your body towards the floor. Return to a standing position.
Knees should not pass the front of the foot.

Weight Shifts, Wall Falls, Balance Recovery (Balance Drills)

	_____ Reps _____ Sets _____X Day _____Hold
31	**Notes:**

SIDE TO SIDE WEIGHT SHIFT
Stand next to stable surface if needed for support.

Keep feet shoulder width apart. Lean from side to side maintaining balance. _May stand in hallway with walls on both sides._
*Advance to using balance pad

	_____ Reps _____ Sets _____X Day _____Hold
32	**Notes:**

FORWARD AND BACKWARDS WEIGHT SHIFTS
Stand next to stable surface if needed for support.

Keep feet shoulder width apart. Lean from body forward and then backwards maintaining balance. _May stand in hallway with wall in front and in back._
 *Advance to using balance pad

	_____ Reps _____ Sets _____X Day _____Hold
33	**Notes:**

SPLIT STANCE WEIGHT SHIFT SIDE TO SIDE
Stand next to stable surface if needed for support.

Stand in a split stance position. Lean side to side maintaining balance. _May stand in hallway with wall on both sides._

	_____ Reps _____ Sets _____X Day _____Hold
34	**Notes:**

SPLIT STANCE WEIGHT SHIFT FORWARD AND BACKWARDS Stand next to stable surface if needed for support.

Stand in a split stance position. Lean forward and backwards maintaining balance. _May stand in hallway with wall in front and in back._

	_____ Reps _____ Sets _____X Day _____Hold
35	**Notes:**

WALL FALLS - FORWARD - BALANCE DRILL

Stand facing wall, a couple feet away from the wall. Slowly and controlled, lean forward towards the wall. Try to control your balance to prevent falling forward. Keep leaning forward gradually until eventually you do lose your balance and fall. Use your arms to catch yourself. Push yourself back upright.

	_____ Reps _____ Sets _____X Day _____Hold
36	**Notes:**

WALL FALLS - LATERAL - BALANCE DRILL

Stand to the side next to a wall, a couple feet away from the wall. Slowly and controlled, lean to the side towards the wall. Try to control your balance to prevent falling sideways. Keep leaning to the side gradually until eventually you do lose your balance and fall. Use your arm to catch yourself. Push yourself back upright.

	_____ Reps _____ Sets _____ X Day _____ Hold
37	**Notes:**

WALL FALLS - BACKWARDS - BALANCE DRILL

Stand facing away from a wall. Slowly and controlled, lean backward towards the wall. Try to control your balance to prevent falling backwards. Keep leaning backwards gradually until eventually you do lose your balance and fall. Use your upper back to catch the fall. Push yourself back upright.

	_____ Reps _____ Sets _____ X Day _____ Hold
38	**Notes:**

WALL FALLS - SINGLE LEG - FORWARD - BALANCE DRILL

Stand on one leg facing a wall, a couple feet away from the wall. Slowly and controlled, lean forward towards the wall. Try to control your balance to prevent falling forward. Keep leaning forward gradually until eventually you do lose your balance and fall. Use your arms to catch yourself. Push yourself back upright.

	_____ Reps _____ Sets _____ X Day _____ Hold
39	**Notes:**

WALL FALLS - SINGLE LEG - LATERAL - BALANCE DRILL

Stand on one leg with a wall a couple feet off to the side of that leg. Slowly and controlled, lean to the side towards the wall. Try to control your balance to prevent falling to the side. Keep leaning gradually towards the wall until eventually you lose your balance and fall. Use your arms to catch yourself. Push yourself back upright.

	_____ Reps _____ Sets _____ X Day _____ Hold
40	**Notes:**

WALL FALLS - SINGLE LEG - MEDIAL - BALANCE DRILL

Stand on one leg with a wall a couple feet off to the opposite side of that leg as shown. Slowly and controlled, lean sideways towards the wall. Try to control your balance to prevent falling to the side. Keep leaning gradually towards the wall until eventually you lose your balance and fall. Use your arms to catch yourself. Push yourself back upright.

	_____ Reps _____ Sets _____ X Day _____ Hold		_____ Reps _____ Sets _____ X Day _____ Hold
41	**Notes:**	**42**	**Notes:**

WALL FALLS - SINGLE LEG - BACKWARDS - BALANCE DRILL

Stand on one leg facing away from a wall. Slowly and controlled, lean backward towards the wall. Try and control your balance to prevent falling backwards. Keep leaning backwards gradually until eventually you do lose your balance and fall. Use your upper back to catch the fall. Push yourself back upright.

FALL LATERAL - STEP RECOVERY
Stand next to stable surface if needed for support.

Start in a standing position with feet apart. Slowly lean to the side and try and prevent losing your balance. Continue to lean to the side until eventually you lose your balance and need to take a step to prevent falling.

	_____ Reps _____ Sets _____ X Day _____ Hold		_____ Reps _____ Sets _____ X Day _____ Hold
43	**Notes:**	**44**	**Notes:**

FALL FORWARD - STEP RECOVERY
Stand next to stable surface if needed for support.

Start in a standing position with feet apart. Slowly lean forward and try and prevent losing your balance. Continue to lean forward until eventually you lose your balance and need to take a step to prevent falling.

FALL BACKWARD - STEP RECOVERY
Stand next to stable surface if needed for support.

Start in a standing position with feet apart. Slowly lean back and try and prevent losing your balance. Continue to lean backwards until eventually you lose your balance and need to take a step to prevent falling.

LEG EXERCISES > BALANCE > RESISTANCE

SOLID GROUND:
1. **Support:** Hold onto chair, counter, sink or another stationary object
2. **No Support:** Stand next to stable surface if needed for support
3. **Resistance:** Add ankle weights on use elastic band for resistance

UNSTABLE SURFACE: Balance pad, Bosu, Half foam roll, Pillow or Other unstable surface
1. **Support:** Hold onto chair, counter or another stationary object.
2. **No Support:** Stand next to stable surface if needed for support.
3. **Resistance:** Add ankle weights on use elastic band for resistance

Peripheral Neuropathy – See beginning of section for Caution on Unstable Surface

	_____ Reps _____ Sets _____X Day _____Hold		_____ Reps _____ Sets _____X Day _____Hold
45	**Notes:**	**46**	**Notes:**

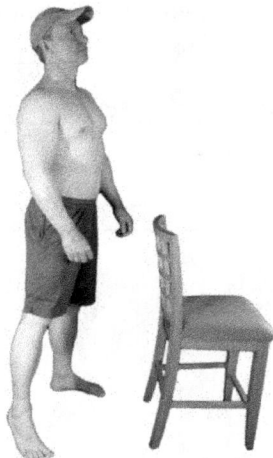

TOE TAP ABDUCTION

Standing upright and move your leg out to the side and tap your toe on the ground. Return to starting position and repeat.

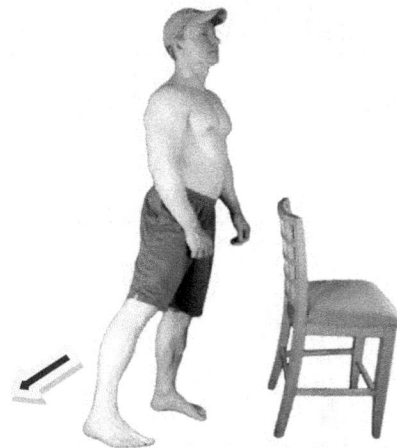

HIP ABDUCTION - STANDING – Can add ankle weights or elastic band.

Standing upright, raise your leg out to the side. Keep your knee straight and maintain your toes pointed forward the entire time. Return to starting position and repeat. Maintain a slow, controlled movement throughout.

	_____ Reps _____ Sets _____ X Day _____ Hold		_____ Reps _____ Sets _____ X Day _____ Hold
47	Notes:	**48**	Notes:

HIP EXTENSION – STANDING - Can add ankle weights or band.

Standing upright, balance on one leg and move your other leg in a backward direction. Do not swing the leg and tighten the buttock at end range. Keep your trunk stable and without arching or bending forward during the movement. Return to starting position and repeat. Maintain a slow, controlled movement throughout.

HIP FLEXION - STANDING – STRAIGHT LEG RAISE - Can add ankle weights or band.

Standing upright, balance on one leg and lift your other leg forward with a straight knee as shown. Return to starting position and repeat. Maintain a slow, controlled movement throughout.

	_____ Reps _____ Sets _____ X Day _____ Hold		_____ Reps _____ Sets _____ X Day _____ Hold
49	Notes:	**50**	Notes:

HIP / KNEE FLEXION - SINGLE LEG - Can add ankle weights

Standing upright, lift your foot and knee up, set it down. Repeat. Maintain a slow, controlled movement throughout.

STANDING MARCHING- Can add ankle weights

Standing upright, draw up your knee, set it down and then alternate to your other side. Maintain a slow, controlled movement throughout.

	_____ Reps _____ Sets _____X Day _____Hold		_____ Reps _____ Sets _____X Day _____Hold
51	Notes:	**52**	Notes:

HAMSTRING CURL - Can add ankle weights.

Standing upright, balance on one leg while bending the knee of the opposite leg towards the buttocks. Return to starting position and repeat. Maintain a slow, controlled movement throughout.

TOE RAISES - Can add hand weights.

Standing upright, go up on your toes slowly towards the ceiling and then return to the starting position. Maintain a slow, controlled movement throughout.

	_____ Reps _____ Sets _____X Day _____Hold		_____ Reps _____ Sets _____X Day _____Hold
53	Notes:	**54**	Notes:

TOE RAISES IR AND ER - Can add hand weights.

IR (Internal Rotation)
Standing upright, rotate feet/legs inward and go up on your toes slowly towards the ceiling and then return to the starting position. Maintain a slow, controlled movement throughout.
ER (External Rotation)
Standing upright, rotate feet/legs outward and go up on your toes slowly towards the ceiling and then return to the starting position.

ONE LEGGED TOE RAISE - Can add hand weights.

Standing upright and balance on one leg. Go up on your toes on the opposite leg towards the ceiling and then return to the starting position. Maintain a slow, controlled movement throughout.

BOSU – Can use chair for stability

_____ Reps _____ Sets _____ X Day _____ Hold	_____ Reps _____ Sets _____ X Day _____ Hold
55 Notes:	**56** Notes:

SINGLE LEG BALANCE FORWARD

Stand on a Bosu with one leg and maintain your balance. Hold your opposite leg out in front of your body and then return to original position. Maintain a slightly bent knee on the stance side.

SINGLE LEG BALANCE LATERAL

Stand on a Bosu with one leg and maintain your balance. Hold your opposite leg out to the side of your body and then return to original position. Maintain a slightly bent knee on the stance side.

_____ Reps _____ Sets _____ X Day _____ Hold	_____ Reps _____ Sets _____ X Day _____ Hold
57 Notes:	**58** Notes:

SINGLE LEG BALANCE RETRO

Stand on a Bosu Ball with one leg and maintain your balance. Hold your opposite leg back behind your body and then return to original position. Maintain a slightly bent knee on the stance side.

SINGLE LEG STANCE RETROLATERAL

Stand on a Bosu Ball with one leg and maintain your balance. Hold your opposite leg back behind and across your body and then return to original position. Maintain a slightly bent knee on the stance side.

	_____ Reps _____ Sets _____ X Day _____ Hold
59	**Notes:**

SQUAT

While standing and maintaining your balance on a Bosu, squat and return to a standing position. Knees should bend in line with the 2nd toe and not pass the front of the foot.

	_____ Reps _____ Sets _____ X Day _____ Hold
60	**Notes:**

SINGLE LEG SQUAT

While standing and balancing on a Bosu with one leg, bend your knee and lower your body towards the ground. Return to a standing position. Your stance knee should bend in line with the 2nd toe and not pass the front of the foot.

Lunges

	_____ Reps _____ Sets _____ X Day _____ Hold
61	**Notes:**

Starting Position

LUNGE – STATIC

Start in standing position with back leg straight and front leg with flexed/bent knee. Lean forward on front knee keeping knee in line with foot and back leg remaining straight. Return to starting position and repeat for several repetitions and then repeat on opposite side.
*Make sure front knee does not go past the foot.

	_____ Reps _____ Sets _____ X Day _____ Hold
62	**Notes:**

Backward   Starting Position   Forward

LUNGE FORWARD/BACKWARD

Start in standing (_middle picture_).
Backward: Keep one foot planted and step back with the opposite foot. Return to original position - repeat. _Forward:_ Keep one foot planted and step forward with the opposite foot. Return to original position - repeat.

DYNAMIC MOVEMENTS

_____ Reps _____ Sets _____X Day _____Hold	_____ Reps _____ Sets _____X Day _____Hold
63 Notes:	**64** Notes:

FOUR CORNER MARCHING IN PLACE

Marching in place, move your body clockwise stopping at each corner for several seconds and move to the next corner. After completing the square, march counterclockwise.

FOUR CORNER MARCHING IN PLACE WITH HEAD TURNS

With Head and Body Moving Simultaneously
March in place to four corners, as previous exercise (#63). Move your head and body moving simultaneously as you complete the square.
With Head Turn And Then Body Turn.
March in place to four corners, as previous exercise (#63). Turn head and then body as you complete the square.

_____ Reps _____ Sets _____X Day _____Hold	_____ Reps _____ Sets _____X Day _____Hold
65 Notes:	**66** Notes:

WALKING ON HEELS FORWARD AND BACKWARDS – May walk along kitchen counter or wall until feeling steady.

Standing up tall, walk forward on heels. After feeling secure with a forward motion, try walking backwards on heels.

WALKING ON TOES FORWARD AND BACKWARDS – May walk along kitchen counter or wall until feeling steady.

Standing up tall, walk forward on up on toes. After feeling secure with a forward motion, try walking backwards up on toes.

67	_____ Reps _____ Sets _____ X Day _____ Hold Notes:	68	_____ Reps _____ Sets _____ X Day _____ Hold Notes:

TANDEM STANCE AND WALK – FORWARD AND BACKWARDS

Maintaining your balance, stand with one foot directly in front of the other so that the toes of one foot touches the heel of the other. Progress by taking steps with your heel touching your toes with each step.
**Progress by walking backwards with your toe touching your heel with each step. Can also add head turns.

RUNNING MAN

Stand and balance on one leg. Lean forward as you bring your other leg back behind you to tap the floor. Bring the same side arm forward as shown during the movement. Return to starting position and repeat.

69	_____ Reps _____ Sets _____ X Day _____ Hold Notes:	70	_____ Reps _____ Sets _____ X Day _____ Hold Notes:

HOP STICK - FORWARD

Stand on one leg and then hop forward onto the other leg. Maintain your balance the entire time. Increase the difficulty by hoping forward further or higher.

HOP STICK - BACKWARDS

Stand on one leg and then hop backward onto the other leg. Maintain your balance the entire time. Increase the difficulty by hoping back further or higher.

	_____ Reps _____ Sets _____ X Day _____ Hold
71	**Notes:**

MINI LATERAL LUNGE

Step to the side and balance on the leg. Next return to the original position. Repeat in the opposite direction. Your knees should be bent about 30 degrees.

	_____ Reps _____ Sets _____ X Day _____ Hold
72	**Notes:**

SIDE STEPPING – May step along kitchen counter or in hallway for support.

Step to the side continuing for length of room or counter – repeat in opposite direction.

	_____ Reps _____ Sets _____ X Day _____ Hold
73	**Notes:**

HOP STICK - LATERAL

Stand on one leg and then hop to the side onto the other leg. Maintain your balance the entire time. Increase the difficulty by hoping to the side further and higher.

	_____ Reps _____ Sets _____ X Day _____ Hold
74	**Notes:**

SINGLE LEG DEAD LIFT

While standing on one leg, bend forward with arms in front towards the ground as you extend your leg behind you and then return to the original position. Keep your legs straight and maintain your balance the entire time.

_____ Reps _____ Sets _____X Day _____Hold		_____ Reps _____ Sets _____X Day _____Hold
75	**Notes:**	**76**	**Notes:**

CONE TAPS - SINGLE LEG STANCE

Place 3-5 cones or cups around you as shown. Balance on a slightly bent knee. Lower yourself down to tap the top of a cone with your finger. Return to original position and repeat touching a different cone. Advance exercise with smaller cones/cups and or faster speed.

CONE TAPS - SINGLE LEG STANCE - UNSTABLE

Place 3-5 cones or cups around you. Balance on an unstable surface such as a foam pad with a slightly bent knee. Lower yourself down to tap the top of a cone. Return to original position and repeat touching a different cone. Advance exercise with smaller cones/cups and or faster speed.

_____ Reps _____ Sets _____X Day _____Hold		_____ Reps _____ Sets _____X Day _____Hold
77	**Notes:**	**78**	**Notes:**

FIGURE 8 AROUND CONES

Set up 4-8 cones on the floor about 12 inches apart, although can vary to increase or decrease difficulty. Weave in and out of cones and then turn and repeat.

FIGURE 8 AROUND CONES – FOOT OR HAND TAP

Follow #75 figure around 4- 8 cones. To increase difficulty, you can tap each cone with your foot or lean over and tap with your hand.

HALF ROLLER (static and dynamic) – FLAT SIDE UP OR DOWN

	_____ Reps _____ Sets _____X Day _____Hold		_____ Reps _____ Sets _____X Day _____Hold
79	**Notes:**	**80**	**Notes:**

BALANCE DOUBLE LEG STANCE - WIDE

Place a half foam roll on the ground in a side-to-side direction. Stand on the foam roll with your feet spread apart and maintain your balance.

BALANCE DOUBLE LEG STANCE - NARROW

Place a half foam roll on the ground in a side-to-side direction. Stand on the foam roll with your feet together and maintain your balance.

	_____ Reps _____ Sets _____X Day _____Hold		_____ Reps _____ Sets _____X Day _____Hold
81	**Notes:**	**82**	**Notes:**

TANDEM STANCE

Place a half foam roll on the ground in a forward-back direction. Stand on the foam roll in tandem stance (with your heel and toe touching as shown) and maintain your balance.

TANDEM WALK

Place a half foam roll on the ground in a forward-back direction. Stand on the foam roll and begin tandem walking (heel-toe pattern walking as shown). Once you get to the end of the roll, either turn around or tandem walk backward.

	_____ Reps _____ Sets _____X Day _____Hold		_____ Reps _____ Sets _____X Day _____Hold
83	Notes:	84	Notes:

SINGLE LEG STANCE - ABDUCTION

Place a half foam roll on the ground in a side-to-side direction. Balance on one leg and move the opposite leg to the side.

SINGLE LEG STANCE - ABDUCTION

Place a half foam roll on the ground in a forward-back direction. Balance on one leg with the opposite leg to the side.

	_____ Reps _____ Sets _____X Day _____Hold		_____ Reps _____ Sets _____X Day _____Hold
85	Notes:	86	Notes:

SINGLE LEG STANCE – FORWARD KICK

Place a half foam roll on the ground in a forward-back direction. Balance on one leg and move the opposite leg forward.

SINGLE LEG STANCE – HAMSTRING CURL

Place a half foam roll on the ground in a forward-back direction. Balance on one leg and with the opposite leg, bend the knee backwards as shown.

Balance

_____ Reps _____ Sets _____X Day _____Hold	_____ Reps _____ Sets _____X Day _____Hold
87 Notes:	**88** Notes:

SINGLE LEG SQUAT – LEG FORWARD

Place a half foam roll on the ground in a forward-back direction. Balance on one leg with a slight bend in the supporting knee and move the opposite leg forward. Straighten supporting knee and repeat.

SINGLE LEG SQUAT – LEG BACKWARDS

Place a half foam roll on the ground in a forward-back direction. Balance on one leg with a slight bend in the supporting knee and with the opposite leg, move the leg backwards as shown with bent knee. Straighten supporting knee and repeat.

STAIR STEP – _To progress, increase step height_

_____ Reps _____ Sets _____X Day _____Hold	_____ Reps _____ Sets _____X Day _____Hold
89 Notes:	**90** Notes:

TOE TAP OR HEEL PLACEMENT

While standing with both feet on the floor, place one foot on the top of the step. Next, return the foot back to the floor and then repeat with the other leg.
You can either put your foot up for several repetitions or alternate.

PULL UP FOOT TOUCHES ON STEP

Whie standing with both feet on the ground, put one foot on the step. Push through the foot straightening the knee until the opposite foot is off the ground. Lower the foot back to the starting position. Repeat with the opposite foot for several repetitions.

_____ Reps _____ Sets _____X Day _____Hold	_____ Reps _____ Sets _____X Day _____Hold

91 Notes:

ALTERNATING SUSTAINED FOOT TOUCHES ON STEP

Whie standing with both feet on the ground, put one foot on the step. Push through the foot straightening the knee until the opposite foot is also on the step. Step off backwards to the starting position. Repeat with the opposite foot for several repetitions.

92 Notes:

STEP UP AND OVER

Step up onto the step and then onto the ground on the other side. Turn around and repeat.
Repeat several repetitions on one side and then the other or alternate legs.

_____ Reps _____ Sets _____X Day _____Hold	_____ Reps _____ Sets _____X Day _____Hold

93 Notes:

FORWARD SWING THROUGH STEP

Step up onto the step without stopping on the top, swing opposite leg through and onto the floor on the other side.

94 Notes:

SIDE STEPPING

****REPEAT STEPS 89-93 from a side approach****

Agility

EXERCISE Agility/Reactivity/Speed	EXERCISE NUMBER	NOTES
Four Square Drills	1	
Dots	2	
Ladder Drills	3	
Box Drills	4	
Cones	5	
Hurdles	6	

Agility/Reactivity/Speed

According to the Twist Conditioning workbook, "Agility is the ability to link several fundamental movement skills into a multidirectional pattern. Reaction skills are the 'whole body' responsiveness to external stimuli, as well as muscle and joint internal reactivity. Quickness is the ability to explosively initiate movement from a stationary position, as well as shifting the gears of speed". (*Twist, Peter, Twist Agility, Quickness and & Reactivity Workbook, 2009, pg 16*)

Agility is a combination of acceleration, deceleration, coordination, power, strength and dynamic balance. With agility training, always keep your head in a neutral position looking straight ahead no matter which way you turn. "Powerful arm movement during transitional and directional changes is essential in order to reacquire a high rate of speed". (*Brown & Ferrigno, 2005, pp 73-74*)

Agility exercises can be done with cones, hurdles, dots or squares on the floor, box drills, Bosu or ladders. Agility can also be high impact or explosive movements. If you are not comfortable with this in the beginning or have any contraindications, stick with low impact movements. In other words, if you are jumping over hurdles, keep them low to the ground and jump over with one leg leading for low impact and jump with both legs for high impact.

If you are doing box drills or Bosu, please do NOT JUMP off backwards.

AGILITY / SPEED / REACTIVITY

4 Square Drills

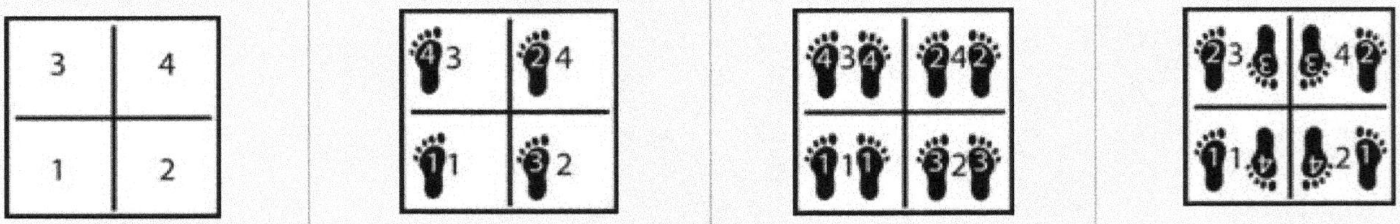

Dots

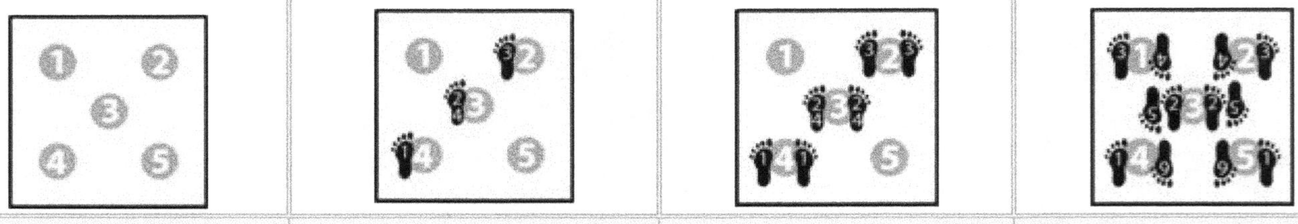

Ladder

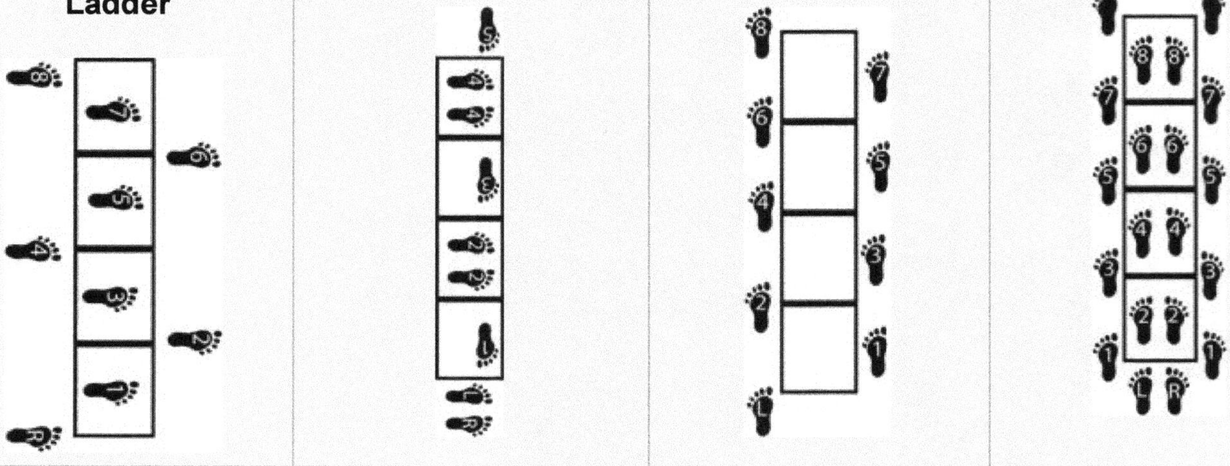

Box Drills – Box should be no higher than the middle of your shin. This can be done on Bosu for balance.

Alt Tap Box With Foot Switch	Down Up Both Feet Together	Quickly Move Side to Side	Down Up Both Feet Together

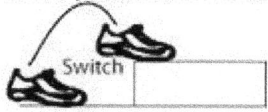

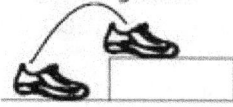

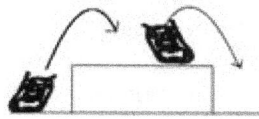

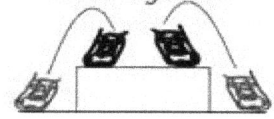

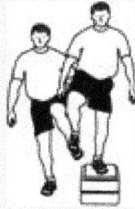

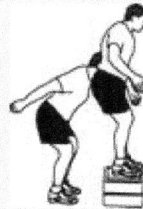

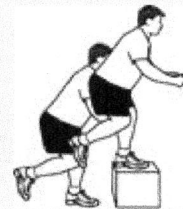

Cones

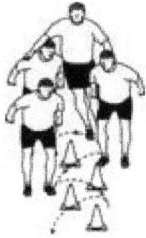

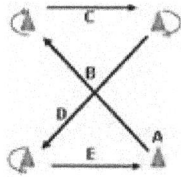

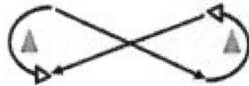

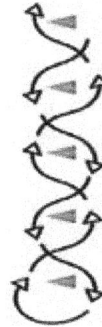

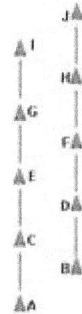

Hurdles – can run or jump over hurdles

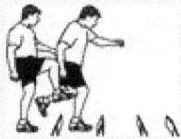

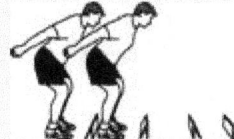

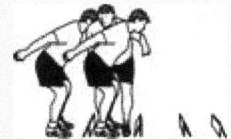

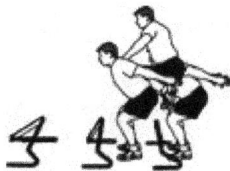

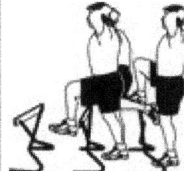

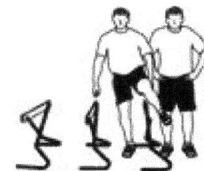

Endurance / Aerobic Capacity

Aerobic - with oxygen: Muscular and Cardiovascular

Many repetitions with sub-maximal weight (weight that is less than the maximum you can lift).

Muscular endurance is the ability of the muscle or group of muscles to sustain repeated contractions against resistance for an extended period of time. This is needed to build muscle. (See *Strengthening*). Cardiovascular endurance is the ability of the heart, lungs and blood vessels to deliver oxygen to working muscles and tissues, as well as the ability of those muscles and tissues to utilize that oxygen. This is needed to help endure long runs or sustained activity, as with biking or running. In short, endurance or aerobic exercises increase the heart rate and respiratory rate.

As far as long-term performance goes, there are two types of muscle fibers that can determine the likelihood of success: slow and fast twitch, which may determine whether you are more likely to be a power-lifter or sprinter (*fast twitch*), or a marathon runner (*slow twitch*). Your ability depends on the distribution of these fibers in the body. In other words, you could have a certain percentage of slow twitch in your biceps, but a different percentage in your quadriceps. There is some controversy over whether you can change the percentage or distribution of these fibers with endurance training or training for a specific event, although you may be able to change the glycolytic capacity.

Type of Fibers	*Slow twitch fibers:* Have a high aerobic capacity and are resistant to fatigue. People that have a higher percentage of slow twitch fibers tend to have better endurance abilities. *Fast twitch fibers:* Contract faster than slow twitch, and thus fatigue faster. People that have a higher percentage of fast twitch fibers tend to have better sprinting or muscle building abilities.

The following research is from the: **MAYO CLINIC**

Mayo Clinic - *https://www.mayoclinic.org/healthy-lifestyle/fitness/in-depth/aerobic-exercise/art-20045541*

Regular aerobic activity, such as walking, bicycling or swimming, can help you live longer and healthier. Need motivation? See how aerobic exercise affects your heart, lungs and blood flow.

How your body responds to aerobic exercise

During aerobic activity, you repeatedly move large muscles in your arms, legs and hips. You'll notice your body's responses quickly.

You'll breathe faster and more deeply. This maximizes the amount of oxygen in your blood. Your heart will beat faster, which increases blood flow to your muscles and back to your lungs.

Your small blood vessels (capillaries) will widen to deliver more oxygen to your muscles and carry away waste products, such as carbon dioxide and lactic acid.

Your body will even release endorphins, natural painkillers that promote an increased sense of well-being.

What aerobic exercise does for your health.

Regardless of age, weight or athletic ability, aerobic activity is good for you. As your body adapts to regular aerobic exercise, you will get stronger and fitter.

Consider the following 10 ways that aerobic activity can help you feel better and enjoy life to the fullest on the next page.

Aerobic activity can help you:

1. **Keep excess pounds at bay**
   Combined with a healthy diet, aerobic exercise helps you lose weight and keep it off.

2. **Increase your stamina**
   You may feel tired when you first start regular aerobic exercise. But over the long term, you'll enjoy increased stamina and reduced fatigue.

3. **Ward off viral illnesses**
   Aerobic exercise activates your immune system in a good way. This may leave you less susceptible to minor viral illnesses, such as colds and flu.

4. **Reduce your health risks**
   Aerobic exercise reduces the risk of many conditions, including obesity, heart disease, high blood pressure, type 2 diabetes, metabolic syndrome, stroke and certain types of cancer.

   Weight-bearing aerobic exercises, such as walking, help decrease the risk of osteoporosis.

5. **Manage chronic conditions**
   Aerobic exercise may help lower blood pressure and control blood sugar. If you have coronary artery disease, aerobic exercise may help you manage your condition.

6. **Strengthen your heart**
   A stronger heart doesn't need to beat as fast. A stronger heart also pumps blood more efficiently, which improves blood flow to all parts of your body.

7. **Keep your arteries clear**
   Aerobic exercise boosts your high-density lipoprotein (HDL), the "good," cholesterol, and lowers your low-density lipoprotein (LDL), the "bad," cholesterol. This may result in less buildup of plaques in your arteries.

8. **Boost your mood**
   Aerobic exercise may ease the gloominess of depression, reduce the tension associated with anxiety and promote relaxation.

9. **Stay active and independent as you age**
   Aerobic exercise keeps your muscles strong, which can help you maintain mobility as you get older. Studies have found that regular physical activity may help protect memory, reasoning, judgment and thinking skills (cognitive function) in older adults and may improve cognitive function in young adults.

10. **Live longer**
    Studies show that people who participate in regular aerobic exercise live longer than those who don't exercise regularly.

Take the first step
Ready to get more active? Great. Just remember to start with small steps. If you've been inactive for a long time or if you have a chronic health condition, get your doctor's OK before you start. When you're ready to begin exercising, start slowly. You might walk five minutes in the morning and five minutes in the evening.
The next day, add a few minutes to each walking session. Pick up the pace a bit, too. Soon, you could be walking briskly for at least 30 minutes a day and reaping all the benefits of regular aerobic activity.

Other options for aerobic exercise could include cross-country skiing, aerobic dancing, swimming, stair climbing, bicycling, jogging, elliptical training or rowing.
(Mayo Clinic - *https://www.mayoclinic.org/healthy-lifestyle/fitness/in-depth/aerobic-exercise/art-20045541*)

Calories

Calorie: A unit of food energy. The word calorie is ordinarily used instead of the more precise, scientific term kilocalorie. A kilocalorie represents the amount of energy required to raise the temperature of a liter of water 1' centigrade at sea level. Technically, a kilocalorie represents 1,000 true calories of energy. *(MedicineNet.com)*

Calories are a measurement tool, like inches or cups. Calories measure the energy a food or beverage provides from the carbohydrate, fat, protein, and alcohol* it contains. Calories give you the fuel or energy you need to work and play – even to rest and sleep! When choosing what to eat and drink, it's important to get the right mix – enough nutrients without too many calories. Paying attention to calories is an important part of managing your weight. The amount of calories you need are different if you want to gain, lose, or maintain your weight. Tracking what and how much you eat, and drink can help you better understand your calorie intake over time. Each person's body may have different needs for calories and exercise. A healthy lifestyle requires balance in the foods you eat, the beverages you drink, the way you do daily activities, adequate sleep, stress management, and in the amount of activity in your daily routine. (*ChooseMyPlate.gov & CDC*)

Example of Activities and Calories Burned (*ChooseMyPlate.gov*)
A 154-pound man who is 5' 10" will use up (burn) about the number of calories listed doing each activity below. Those who weigh more will use more calories; those who weigh less will use fewer calories. The calorie values listed include both calories used by the activity and the calories used for normal body functioning during the activity time.

EXAMPLE	Approximate calories used (burned) by a 154-pound man	
MODERATE physical activities:	**In 1 hour**	**In 30 minutes**
Hiking	370	185
Light gardening/ yard work	330	165
Dancing	330	165
Golf (walking and carrying clubs)	330	165
Bicycling (less than 10 mph)	290	145
Walking (3.5 mph)	280	140
Weight training (general light workout)	220	110
Stretching	180	90
VIGOROUS physical activities:	**In 1 hour**	**In 30 minutes**
Running/ jogging (5 mph)	590	295
Bicycling (more than 10 mph)	590	295
Swimming (slow freestyle laps)	510	255
Aerobics	480	240
Walking (4.5 mph)	460	230
Heavy yard work (chopping wood)	440	220
Weightlifting (vigorous effort)	440	220
Basketball (vigorous)	440	220

References

Also, Some Good Books, Websites & DVD'

ACE Idea Fitness Journal: *Martina M. Cartwright, PhD, RD http://www.ideafit.com/fitness-library/protein-today-are-consumers-getting-too-much-of-a-good-thing?ACE_ACCESS=ebec6bcf61abff08f7b1d8b27c555758*

ACE Senior Fitness Manual, *American Council on Exercise* (2014)

American Physical Therapy Association, (APTA), 2007. *Basic Science for Animal Physical Therapy: Canine, 2nd edition*

Arleigh J Reynolds, DVM, PhD - *www.absasleddogracing.org.uk/newgang/src/gangline/role.htm*

Australian Institute of Sports - *http://www.ausport.gov.au*

BodyBuilder.com

Brown & Ferrigno, (2005). *Training for Speed, Agility and Quickness*, Champaign, IL: Human Kinetics.

Bryant, C & Green, D, editors (2003), *Ace Personal Trainer Manual, 3rd ed.*, San Diego, CA: American Council on Exercise (ACE)

ChooseMyPlate.gov

Examine.com

ExRx.net

Feher & Szunyoghy (1996). *Cyclopedia Anatomicae,* Tess Press

Gillette, R (2002). Temperature Regulation of the Dog. Retrieved June 2011 from *http://www.sportsvet.com/11Nwsltr.PDF*

Gillette, R (2008). *Feeding the Canine Athlete for Optimal Performance.* Retrieved September 25, 2008 from *www.sports vet.com/Art3.html.*

Glucose (Wikipedia) - *http://en.wikipedia.org/wiki/Glucose*

Glycemic Index (Wikipedia) - *http://en.wikipedia.org/wiki/Glycemic_index*

LiveStrong.com

Mayo Clinic - *https://www.mayoclinic.org/healthy-lifestyle/fitness/in-depth/aerobic-exercise/art-20045541*

MedicineNet.com

Myofascial Release: (Wikipedia) - https://en.wikipedia.org/wiki/Myofascial_release

Rikli, Roberta and Jones, Jessie (2013) *Senior Fitness Test Manual, 2nd Ed,*

Strength Training: (Wikipedia) *http://en.wikipedia.org/wiki/Strength_training*

Twist, Peter (2009). *Twist Agility, Quickness and & Reactivity Workbook.* British Columbia: Twist Conditioning, Inc. University of Maryland Medical Center.com

Workout Australia

Thank You to:

My Husband
Model
For his support through my battle with cancer and while writing this and previous books.
Also, for the patience and hours he put in modeling for this book.

My Daughter
For giving me artistic inspiration and providing artwork for my previous books.

My Grandchildren
Just Because

God
For giving me the strength to overcome cancer and the wisdom to write these books.

Certifications, Continuing Education and License

Physical Therapist Assistant – L/PTA – 30 years in both Home Therapy and Short-Term Rehab facilities

ACE Certified Personal Trainer – CPT
- o **Functional Training Specialist**
- o **Therapeutic Exercise Specialist**
- o **Senior Fitness Specialist**
- o **Nutrition and Fitness Specialist**

©Klose Education
- o **Certified Lymphedema Therapist – CLT**
- o **Strength After Breast Cancer – Strength ABC**
- o **Breast Cancer Rehabilitation**

©Cancer Exercise Specialist Institute – CETI
- o **Cancer Exercise Specialist – CES**
- o **Breast Cancer Recovery BOSU(R) Specialist Advanced Qualification**
- o **Pilates Mat Certificate**

©MedFit
- o **Medical Fitness Specialist**
- o **Parkinson's Disease Fitness Specialist**
- o **Arthritis Fitness Specialist**

©Pink Ribbon Program

©The BioMechanics Method - Corrective Exercise Specialist

©ISSA - DNA-Based Fitness Coach

www.ingramcontent.com/pod-product-compliance
Lightning Source LLC
Chambersburg PA
CBHW052110020426
42335CB00021B/2707